YOUR FIFTY-PLUS BODY—A COOK'S TOUR

You look in the mirror now, and you look a bit different than you did at thirty or forty. You call it age. And time can alter your looks, no denying it. And yet, too often, what we take as signs of aging are really signs of poor nutrition.

I can hear you now. "Poor nutrition!" you laugh. "*Over*abundance is my problem." But wait. What are you getting in your meals and snacks? Do you realize that your nutritional needs are changing, now that you're fifty or more? That, now, even a seemingly healthful diet can accelerate the aging process?

You can help ensure that these physical changes don't become health worries. Diet is your vehicle. While a preventive diet can't *guarantee* you'll never have a health problem, it can, in many cases, mean the difference between health and illness. On the Palm Beach Diet—the ultimate preventive plan—you protect your health while you lose weight. You also protect your health with exercise.

Now let's turn to the nitty-gritty ingredients of the diet that can make you look and feel years younger . . .

THE PALM BEACH LONG-LIFE DIET

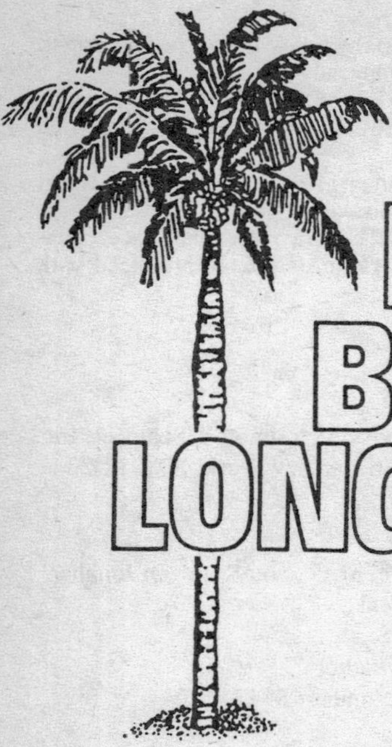

THE PALM BEACH LONG-LIFE DIET

E. JOAN BARICE, M.D.
WITH KATHLEEN JONAH

PUBLISHED BY POCKET BOOKS NEW YORK

Grateful acknowledgment is made to the following for permission to reprint from previously published materials:

Chart of food additives on pp. 195-207 © 1983 Center for Science in the Public Interest, 1501 16th Street, N.W., Washington, D.C. 20036.

Guidelines for restaurant dining on pp. 182-185 © American Heart Association. Reproduced with permission.

Exercise text on pp. 213-235 © The Travelers Insurance Companies, 1 Tower Square, Hartford, Conn. 06115. Reproduced with permission.

POCKET BOOKS, a division of Simon & Schuster, Inc.
1230 Avenue of the Americas, New York, N.Y. 10020

Exercise drawings by Lamont O'Neal

Published by arrangement with the author
Library of Congress Catalog Card Number: 84-22127

ISBN: 0-671-61211-5

First Pocket Books printing February, 1986

10 9 8 7 6 5 4 3 2 1

Printed in the U.S.A.

Contents

Foreword by Joseph Jordan Eller, M.D. ix

Introducing the Palm Beach Diet xiii

PART ONE:

New-Age Prescriptions for Well-Being

1. It's Not Too Late 3
2. A Diet for a New Age 13
3. America's Aged Elite—and Your Elite Body 23
4. Palm Beach Health Dividends—Vitamins and Minerals 32
5. Palm Beach Health Dividends—Biochemical Balances 50
6. Losing (Weight) Gracefully 60

PART TWO:

The 21 Days That Will Change Your Life

7. The Palm Beach Diet 69
8. The Palm Beach Diet—Easy Week 89
9. The Palm Beach Diet—"The Breakers" Week 100
10. Questions and Answers 116
11. How to Pull It Off 143

PART THREE:
Health Ammunition for the Mature Years

12. How to Keep It Off 159
13. More New-Age Survival Tactics 186
14. Fifty-Plus Exercise 213
15. Sex, and a Note on Stress 236
16. The Bottom Line on Prevention 243

Appendix: Medications, Drugs and Diet 261

Bibliography 277

Acknowledgments 297

About the Authors 299

Note to the Reader

The Palm Beach Long-Life Diet is intended as a preventive diet against common diseases associated with aging. By encouraging weight loss, this diet can help lower the risk of obesity-related illness and control some cases of high blood pressure and diabetes. It will lower cholesterol levels in some individuals. It will help prevent or slow the natural progression of a number of other health complaints.

The Palm Beach Long-Life Diet cannot reverse existing disease, however, with the exception, in *some* cases, of those cited above.

Before you go on the Palm Beach Long-Life Diet, check with your doctor. This is vitally important. Overweight, especially at the age of fifty or more, is often accompanied by a health condition or two that may require medical attention. Some people intending to diet may have high blood pressure or diabetes, for example, without being aware of it. Both conditions respond to weight loss and dietary treatment, but they require medical treatment as well.

While you're following the Palm Beach Long-Life Diet, continue to take any medication that has been prescribed for you. The Palm Beach Long-Life Diet is *not* a substitute for medication. At a later date, after finishing the diet, you may require a lower dose of medication; however, the decision to alter your prescription must be left to your doctor.

Foreword

A whole generation of people over fifty is discovering the joy of fitness. They are learning that they can be in far better shape now than they were ten or even twenty years ago. All that may be needed are the tools of good diet and exercise, and a positive attitude.

Nowhere is the idea of optimal health more evident than here in Palm Beach, where living well is *de rigueur.* I follow many of the Palm Beach Long-Life Diet's principles myself, including an early morning swim or a brisk walk, and I am healthy and vigorous after being in the active practice of medicine for over fifty years. My mornings are now devoted to a busy practice specializing in skin diseases and skin surgery. In the afternoon, as president and director general of the Pan American Medical Association for the past twenty-five years, I play an active role in furthering the continuing education of physicians in the thirty-one Western Hemisphere nations.

There is more to my life than work, however. I attend many social events in Palm Beach, where I see people older than myself dancing to beat the band! Such physical activity, in combination with a wisely chosen diet, can create an enviable zest for living in those over fifty.

Little did most of us realize, back before "diet" had become a household word, that by choosing the right foods, we could avoid the nutritional risk factors of chronic disease. What a terrifically important and useful fact this is! By eating the right kinds and combinations of fats, as an example, the cholesterol level of the blood can be kept in the ranges that reduce the risk of heart attack. Adequate intake of high fiber foods such as vegetables and legumes, fruits and cereals may help reduce the risk of colon cancer.

Aware of accumulating knowledge within the nutritional sciences, I was enthusiastic when the notion of a health plan for the mature individual first was put forward. Having long known Dr. Barice and her fine work in public health, I had no doubt that this remarkable woman could interpret the latest medical findings for a wide audience. I have seen Dr. Barice organize local programs on health maintenance, alcohol and drug addiction, and nutrition. She serves on the faculty of the University of Miami Medical School and is an advisor on matters of health and public health administration to U.S. Congressman Tom Lewis. A graduate of Stanford University Medical School with a Master's degree in Public Health from Harvard, Dr. Barice is board certified in Internal and Preventive Medicines. The Palm Beach Community awarded her its Distinguished Professional Woman in Leadership honor in 1984.

Given her unparalleled reputation for excellence, I was certain that she would bring professionalism and warmth to the task of developing this over-fifty diet plan. I was not disappointed. The Palm Beach Long-Life Diet deserves the praise that has been heaped upon it from top authorities in the field.

It's quite natural that as an individual matures, he or she takes a keener interest in health. This generally is a positive development. Occasionally, however, this concern manifests itself in anxiety or fear. How very much more life-affirming to start now—at fifty, sixty or whatever age—to take steps toward mature health. Dr. Barice's optimism on this point is contagious.

In my opinion, this book is the most scientific to date in the area of diet and nutrition. Read Dr. Barice's fine book closely. You will discover how to live a longer and better life.

JOSEPH JORDAN ELLER, M.D.
Palm Beach, Florida

Introducing the Palm Beach Diet

When was the last time you looked in the mirror—and actually smiled?

a. Last week
b. Last year
c. During the Eisenhower administration

What haven't you done since you can't remember when?

a. Danced the Lindy Hop
b. Stayed out until dawn
c. Seen your toes

You've joked about it—despaired over it. And finally tried to live with it. But it whittles away at your pride; it makes you feel older than your years. I'm talking about *fat,* of course. When you're overweight, life can feel like the last plane left for Fort Lauderdale hours ago, and you're stuck in a snow drift.

You've tried diets, you say. Nothing works. At least not for very long. And it's true—or at least it was, before *the Palm Beach Long-Life Diet*. This comprehensive plan is designed to help people fifty or older attain a youthful, slimmer shape. Safely—triumphantly—and for a lifetime, not just for a few weeks. I'm thrilled to share my program with you. Here in Florida, the Palm Beach Long-Life Diet has changed lives. It can do the same for you.

What is so special about *this* diet over all the others you've tried? Perhaps most important, it can improve your health as it improves your shape: It is carefully formulated to provide those nutrients you need now, at fifty and over, to maintain optimal health. The diet also helps your mature system achieve ideal biochemical balances, and it champions the work of the immune system. And it does all this without feeling like a "medical" diet: Palm Beach residents have a tradition of fine, slimming cuisine upon which this diet is based. It will utterly spoil you! In short, the Palm Beach Long-Life Diet reinvents what it means and what it takes to lose weight.

This unique plan is a Florida "natural" in many ways. Florida boasts more people over age fifty, per capita, than any other state. Our Sunshine State also embraces some of the wealthiest communities in the country. Many residents make a priority of bristling good health, and the slim "well-heeled" look—it is said that diets are followed as closely here as the Dow Jones Industrial Average! In fact, I have yet to meet anyone here in Palm Beach County (along the Gold Coast towns of Jupiter Island, Singer Island, Palm Beach, Boca Raton and Delray Beach) who is *not* interested in a good, healthy and long life.

Southern Florida is a focal point for the same health concerns of people in their middle-to-mature years everywhere. Our adult population scans the same reports that you do—on the "wonders" of this or that nutrient; on life-prolonging techniques; on new diet programs. My mature patients ask me to help them discriminate between sound and dangerous diets and to sort out life-extension quackery from reliable advice. As a former public-health administrator, and as a practicing physican who is board certified in Preventive Medicine and Internal Medicine, I am often called to the front line in the local diet fervor. Local legislators consult me on public health policy. I've been guest and hostess on many television and radio programs that deal with health. I speak to groups on behalf of the Palm Beach County Medical Society. And I can vouch firsthand: Nowhere is the public more eager for accurate, current and useful information than in the area of diet and health.

This is another important aspect of the diet: You'll discover many fascinating and helpful tips in the pages ahead—pointers that help you decode the superabundance of new information issuing out of nutrition research. You'll also find pointers which will emancipate you from some hidebound myths about dieting. I believe this is a state-of-the-art plan, and one that answers the special needs of almost everyone fifty or more.

Before you slip off to the sunny pages ahead, a word about the diet itself: It is enticing. You will find it a stunning departure from dreary "diet plates." This, after all, is Palm Beach, home to some of the world's best private and club chefs. On the diet (referred to in shorthand as the Palm Beach Diet throughout these pages), you'll enjoy a number of menus and recipes created especially for you by executive chef Karl Ronaszeki, of the world-famous Palm Beach hotel, The Breakers.

Palm Beachers have learned how to stay lean and sleek while indulging in candle-lit patio dinners, elegant lawn parties on the intracoastal, hors d'oeuvre on the yacht, and champagne and strawberries at the polo matches. We boast a fabulous—but portable—approach to diet that you can follow regardless of where you live. Everything you'll need is available in your hometown. And for those of you who want to diet with as little fuss and time preparation as possible, there's an "Easy Week" plan that's as streamlined as it is healthful.

I think you're going to love what lies ahead. My patients tell me that the Palm Beach Diet is the first plan they've tried that they actually have enjoyed. They say it's a gourmet spree, without being fussy. That makes me glow—and then gloat, too, because *I* know it also is serious medicine, based on authoritative research in nutrition and aging. It is truly the renaissance diet of the 1980s.

Along with the diet, you'll find a few preliminary chapters illuminating the importance of sound nutrition once you reach fifty or more. You'll discover what you can expect from your body, too. Based on recent research, all of this information is easy to read and quite fascinating. It also is essential to the healthy, well-informed person, so don't bypass these chapters in your haste to get to the diet. If you have a better understanding of how the Palm Beach Diet works, you'll be better prepared to see that it does!

The later chapters of this book also are a "know-how" bonanza. You'll learn that exercise—a vital adjunct to any diet—can be enjoyable and safe *at any age.* I strongly recommend that you follow the Palm Beach Diet's step-by-step exercise advice as you diet—with your own doctor's blessing and supervision, of course. You'll also learn to become a discriminating food buyer: I don't want you taken for a ride by "all-natural" promises, or thrown for a loop by misleading claims. You'll come to recognize what kinds of nutritional supplements are a boon and which are bunk. And, finally, the pages ahead will show you how to *maintain* your weight loss, and make the principles and the spirit of the Palm Beach Diet yours for a lifetime.

It's all here for you, and I'll be escorting you at every step. Enjoy!

E. JOAN BARICE, M.D., M.P.H.
Palm Beach Gardens, Florida

PART ONE

New-Age Prescriptions for Well-Being

CHAPTER 1

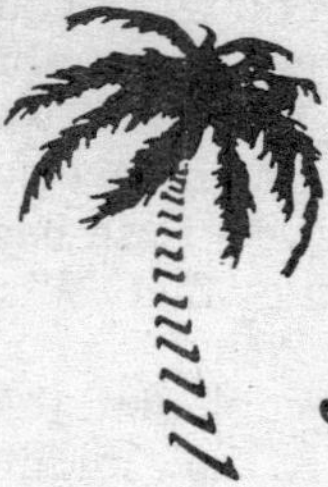

It's Not Too Late

"It's too late for me!" is the classic response from my mature patients when I suggest they should lose weight. Most of them have experienced a slow, creeping weight gain beginning in their middle years, despite sporadic dieting. The typical American pattern is to gain one pound a year between the ages of twenty-five and fifty. This means that by the age of fifty, many Americans are roughly twenty-five pounds overweight!

Once-firm contours shift, too: Accumulating weight tends to go south with age—and I don't mean to Miami. I mean to the stomach and hips. These patients haven't touched their toes—or a bathing suit—in years. As they put it time and time again, how can they begin to dream of a slim shape *at their age?*

They can. You can. Good looks and vitality aren't assigned expiration dates; you get stamped "over the hill" only if you choose to let your body and your health slide.

Perhaps you deny that your looks matter at this stage of life. That denial, though, probably is a little white lie you've decided to tell yourself. Many people are quick to lean on that totem to self-deception: "It's silly to care about appearance at my age." As if there were a cutoff point at which we stop caring about ourselves—as if pride takes an early retirement! The truth is, whatever your age, you feel good when you take care of yourself.

"Letting yourself go" is something you should confine to the dance floor. You don't want to do it with your looks or your life. Aging in fact is an invitation to do just the opposite—to make a fresh beginning—to love yourself. What do I mean by that? What does love have to do with losing weight? Plenty.

After fifty, most people find that the work and family pressures that marked their middle years ease. Activities become more a matter of choice, less a daily itinerary of obligations. There's time now to indulge a few private goals and desires.

So indulge away! It's your turn. Make your fresh start by learning to be good to yourself. If you're in relatively good health and free of chronic illness, it's not too late to shape up *and* start to build nutritional safeguards into your diet. It's not too late to put pride back into your step.

When you say it's too late for you, by the way, you're admitting some pretty old-fashioned ideas about growing older. It's as if you're saying that your middle-to-mature years can't be satisfying and vital. You're likening life to a washed-out ballgame—and a fiftieth or sixtieth birthday to a rainout in which you pack up your dreams and go home after the fifth inning.

But that's *not* what aging has to be!

As you'll see in the next chapters, today's "young old" are reinventing what it means to be older. Educated, active, involved, they promise to be a whole new generation of "senior citizens" in coming years—a group to which the clichés of old age no longer apply. They've lived through unprecedented scientific and social change; they've shaped the most prosperous years in the country's history. Women in their fifties and sixties today were the most fertile of any generation before them; many went back to school and to work after the children left the nest. My point in this is that never before has a generation of older Americans been as sophisticated or as forward-thinking. It's certainly not too late for you. In fact, you're at the threshold of a dynamic era for over-fifties.

This aptitude for vitality, and the time you now have to spend on yourself are wonderful gifts. Use them and invest in your future well-being. Let the Palm Beach Diet be your starting point. It will show you how to have a more youthful physique—and its attendant sparkle.

Before you get started, though, let's run through some of the hesitations you may have about starting yet another diet. These are the rationalizations that you may use to excuse yourself from dieting again, especially when you're feeling discouraged. *Don't believe them*—they're cop-outs. I'll explain why.

It's-Too-Late-for-Me Excuse #1

> *"Come on. Me, at my age, on a diet? Why should I deny myself the occasional treat and splurge. I've worked hard all my life, and now it's time for me to take it easy. I've earned that dessert!"*

I agree that you shouldn't have to give up the occasional treat. You *have* worked hard; you do deserve more than skeleton rations. The Palm Beach Diet is an enjoyable way of life, not a punishment; that's why you'll have, at appropriate intervals and combined with other nutritious foods, "treats" like ice cream, pasta and pancakes. You're given a snack each day—for reasons of appetite control and medical soundness.

How can you get away with such undiet-like food? Two reasons. First, the bottom line of the Palm Beach Diet is balance: You can have linguine tonight—if you have it with fish and a vegetable—and not the garlic bread too. The following morning you don't have bread—you save it for lunch, with a seafood salad, perhaps. In other words, you *space* your treats; you don't eliminate them. You surround them with less calorie-dense foods so by the end of the day, you've had your cake and eaten it too—without straying out of bounds and topping the scales.

I know that at your age you have some food habits that are very much a part of your lifestyle. These are difficult to break. So don't break them, just *balance* them.

It's my observation that people over fifty think about food a bit more than younger people. They appreciate that food is a real pleasure in life and that meals are an especially important part of every day. Also, for these people social activities often center on food; meals shared at home or in a restaurant provide important opportunities to enjoy old friends and to get to know new ones better.

Food can also be a problem in later years. You may be at home more—within tempting proximity of the refrigerator. If you're alone a great deal or generally dissatisfied with your life, food can fill a pleasure gap—and the pounds pile on.

What happens then? You find yourself in a tug-of-war between your good intentions on one hand . . . and a slew of psychological diet-slayers on the other hand. You've got noble diet goals—but the pleasure, comfort and friendship associated with eating remain powerful incentives to wander from boring and contrived diet plans.

Here's a typical "I'm on a diet" scenario:

"We're all going out tonight to Giorgio's Italian restaurant. Won't you join us?"

Sigh. Expletive. Gulp. You don't want to miss out, but *you're on a diet:* "Sorry, I'd love to go. But I'm on a diet, and tonight it calls for three green beans and six grapes."

"Just have the antipasto and a glass of wine."

"I'm not allowed the antipasto. I'm not allowed wine."

In other words, you're not allowed to enjoy food! And you'll soon be off that diet because it bore little resemblance to your normal eating style.

Most diets fail to recognize this aspect of the mature lifestyle. Restaurant meals and dinners with friends are luxuries you can afford now. Diets that limit you to an arbitrary and contrived regimen rob you of these psychological and social pleasures. But on the Palm Beach Diet, you'll have a "normal" diet pattern, and still lose weight.

It's-Too-Late-for-Me Excuse #2

> *"I'm afraid of diets, now that I'm over fifty. I hear stories about people becoming ill on diets, and even of a few deaths linked to weight-loss plans. I'm not as young and resilient as I used to be. I'm afraid that dieting will harm, rather than benefit, my health."*

Good point. Many of the quick weight-loss plans that have made headlines prey on the fantasies of the millions of overweight Americans who desperately want to be trim. Many of these diets are hazardous to your health. They deprive you of calories, and the nutrients your body needs to maintain and repair organs, to nourish cells and to keep the immune system functioning optimally. Some people have become ill, and a few have died on these diets!

Generally, dieting does stress the mature body more than it does the younger body. Your system *is* less resilient than it once was. Just as the common cold or the flu can be more devastating and have broader consequences as you age, a capricious diet can take more of a health toll on the mature individual.

This is where the Palm Beach Diet differs from almost every diet you've tried to date: It's as concerned with a healthy and long life as it is with your looks. The best of medical and nutritional research has been brought to bear in its recommendations. It can actually help the body repair itself, maintain its functioning and prevent the premature onset of many chronic diseases. The Palm Beach Diet is based on the most recent nutritional research and as a result it provides all the nutrients you need to make you strong and healthy and to maintain the immune system.

It's-Too-Late-for-Me Excuse #3

> *"It happens every time I diet. I lose some weight, but then I gain it all back. What makes the Palm Beach Diet different?"*

"Weight rebound" is a problem for many dieters. In fact, most people who lose weight do gain it back; diet success is followed by diet failure. This is a very frustrating problem—one that many diet plans ignore.

The main reason for weight rebound is simple: Pounds pile back on when, after dieting and achieving your weight goal, you revert to old eating habits. On the Palm Beach Diet, you'll lose weight and learn how to *maintain* your new, slimmer figure. This is vital.

In some cases, returned *water* weight is the post-dieter's undoing. When you follow a crash diet, you may lose more water than fat. The low-carbohydrate diets are popular cases in point; weight-loss is often rapid, but as soon as you resume a normal and balanced diet, you begin once again to retain water normally, too. You just can't win on a crash diet: As soon as you go off it, you regain the weight you lost. And if you stay on it, it's possible to harm your health.

Many diets are noted for being rigorous and very

low-calorie. And what do you suppose happens after a week or two of calorie deprivation? You can guess: The body rebels, and the dieter swings to the opposite extreme—overeating. As quickly as they left, unwanted pounds come home.

The interesting theory behind this is that the body, denied its usual calorie allotment, acts to make up for lost calories. When you lose weight suddenly, the urge to dig into an entire coffee cake or a pint of ice cream is biological. The brain appears to signal the appetite centers to initiate feelings of hunger. It's as if the body is trying to sabotage your attempts to upset its fat status!

While no diet can completely eliminate the postdiet urge to indulge, some are better at it than others. The Palm Beach Diet is one of the best, because it does not deprive you of too many calories or delicious foods.

On the Palm Beach Diet, you won't feel a desperate need to recoup lost calories because it maintains weight loss at a moderate pace. At fifty or more, you do *not* want to take off weight rapidly; doing so can jeopardize your health *and* make you especially vulnerable to food-bingeing. You want a satisfying rate of loss that doesn't risk biochemical trauma. I'll explain more about weight-loss "pace" in Chapter 6. For now, know that the Palm Beach Diet will help you lose weight *and keep weight off.*

It's-Too-Late-for-Me Excuse #4

> *"I'm sixty years old. I'm afraid that if I lose weight, I'll wrinkle more. I'd rather be a little chubby-cheeked than look like a bloodhound . . ."*

This is a special concern for men and women who diet later in life. The skin becomes less resilient with age and doesn't shrink back as readily when you lose weight. This can result in a certain amount of looseness to the skin. What has happened? Where fat once was stored—just beneath the skin—there is now a pocket of empty space!

Rapid weight loss is the culprit here. Wrinkling and sagging occur when fat disappears faster than the skin can react. Then, too, lost fat may be replaced by body fluids during rapid weight loss. This produces a bloated look.

Losing weight at a moderate pace is your best defense. A moderate rate of weight loss—á la the Palm Beach Diet—allows the skin to accommodate change better. The Palm Beach Diet also helps combat this problem by reducing salt intake and recommending regular exercise; both reduce water accumulation. But most important, the diet favors less wrinkling because it gives the body more time to adapt as you lose fat.

It's-Too-Late-for-Me Excuse #5

> *"Sometimes I can't get to the grocery store for days. I prefer convenience foods for this reason. I live alone, too, and don't like preparing fussy meals."*

On the Palm Beach Diet, most frozen food is fine. Frozen vegetables, for example, can be as nutritious as fresh—even more so in some cases. Many so-called "fresh" vegetables and fruits spend two to three days in transit to the grocery store, and then time in the bin, or on the shelf, too. During that time, they are continually losing nutritional value. Frozen vegetables, meanwhile, remain nearly as nutritious as they were the moment of freezing. If you can't find "fresh" foods or you do your marketing just once a week or so, opt for frozen.

Canned foods, however, are generally a poor third choice. Most are doused in salt and/or sugar. In most cases, I recommend frozen foods over canned foods.

Want more convenience? You've got it. The Palm

Beach Diet does allow some foods that contain preservatives. Some preservatives are a boon for the infrequent shopper, as they prevent food from spoiling quickly once it's brought home.

No, I'm *not* committing health food heresy by recommending preserved foods. Preservatives aren't all hazardous. In fact, preliminary research suggests that some chemical preservatives—such as BHT—may help protect against some cancers. In Chapter 13, I explain which chemical food additives are good, bad and indifferent. Right now, though, feel free to use preservative-containing breads, cheeses, oils and ice creams.

Another Palm Beach plus is the convenience of commercially prepared food. Some ready-made items are written into the diet. For example, you're allowed to substitute up to two meals each week with a commercially prepared frozen diet meal—if you choose to. These low-calorie frozen entrees are very popular *because* they're convenient; they're basically good nutrition, and low in fat, which makes them some of the best "fast foods" around.

Inconvenience is no excuse on the Palm Beach Diet.

It's-Too-Late-for-Me Excuse #6

> *"You've overlooked the big reason I needn't sweat out a diet. Admit it. It's normal to gain weight as you grow older, isn't it?"*

Sorry. It's not biologically ordained that somehow people gain weight as they age. In fact, you should lose weight as you grow older! Why? As you age, you lose muscle—and muscle is weighty stuff. The Palm Beach Diet includes exercise as a health-promoting adjunct to the diet to help prevent this loss of muscle and strength while you lose weight.

You think it's normal to gain weight with age because

that's what you see around you. As I said before, the typical American pattern is to gain one pound each year between the ages of twenty-five and fifty. That's both unnecessary and unhealthy. Think for a moment: How many obese older people do you see day-to-day on the street and in the marketplace who lead active lives? Very few, for the sad and obvious reason that extreme overweight and age almost guarantee disability. It's definitely not natural—nor is it desirable—to gain weight with age. While this area of ideal weight and aging is controversial—some observers have recently suggested that weight gain with age is normal and healthy—the bulk of research strongly links a slimming and a healthy diet with longevity.

Too late for you? No way! Excuses enough, I'd say. Now on to *positive* thinking!

CHAPTER 2

A Diet for a New Age

If you're fifty or more, you're among one of the fastest growing segments of the U.S. population—more than one of every four Americans today is fifty-plus. One of every four! And this increase in the older population is expected to keep snowballing through to the year 2000 and beyond. Maturity has come of age—like an avalanche—in America.

The country's population is graying because we're living longer: If you were sixty-five in 1960, for example, you could have expected to live another 14.3 years, on average, according to the National Center for Health Statistics life tables. But in 1978, as a sixty-five-year-old, you could have expected to live another 16.3 years. In just two decades, in other words, the life expectancy for sixty-five-year-olds advanced two full years. If you're fifty *now*, on average, your life expectancy is another 24.6 years if you're male; 30.5 years if you're female. Even at the age of eighty-five today, you've got on average another 6.4 years to look forward to!

If that news weren't happy enough, some researchers feel that these government projections are low. A 1983 meeting of the American Association for the Advancement of Science predicted a continued *sharp rise* in life expectancy.

A recent Census Bureau report on aging in America contains more happy surprises: In the coming years, the fastest growing segment of the older population won't be the fifty-ish "young old," but those eighty-five and over! The mortality rate for people over eighty-five is decreasing especially fast. Some scientists see these trends as indications that we're approaching a maximum life expectancy of about ninety-five years!

So the good news is that we're living longer. It's not the whole picture, however. Living longer does not necessarily mean you'll live a better or healthier life. *In fact, the Census Bureau reports that while the death rate is dropping, the disability rate is climbing.*

Many older Americans now find themselves in the precarious position of surviving into old age, but with conditions that limit their mobility and vigor. Many of these illnesses are "chronic"—progressive and long-lasting conditions. Heart disease, cancer, diabetes, hypertension (high blood pressure) and visual and hearing impairments are the biggest contributors to the recent increase in disabilities.

There's more startling news here, too. The age at which chronic health problems manifest themselves is getting younger. According to the National Institute on Aging—part of the federal government's prestigious National Institutes of Health—*rates of illness, particularly chronic illness, are increasing most rapidly among the group aged forty-five to sixty-four.* By age sixty-five, most people have well-established illnesses.

What do these statistics mean to you? They mean that your chance of living into your seventies or eighties and beyond has never been better—but so is your chance of having to cope with a serious health condition in later life. It means that surgical and pharmacological advances are keeping us alive longer, and that medical science is curbing "acute" diseases such as infections. But this trend also reveals that we are still stymied by many chronic diseases.

This doesn't mean, though, that you can't minimize *your* risks by acting on what we now know about preventive medicine. We have documented evidence, for instance, that lifestyle choices including diet, exercise, stress reduction and not smoking do more to keep you healthy than all other health care measures put together!

A healthy lifestyle is without question the best preventive medicine. It's the ammunition you need *now* as you enter the years in which chronic illness can turn a satisfying life into an endurance contest.

The Palm Beach Diet is precisely the preventive measure you need. Diet can affect how long you live; diet can also affect how *well* you live. *It has been estimated that one-third to one-half of the health problems of the aged are in part diet-related. It is well-established that diet can modify the aging process.* That says it all. Now it's up to you to take a super-healthy plan like the Palm Beach Diet and put it to work for you. You *can* lower your risk of contracting chronic illness. I see the wonderful results every day in patients who take part in my preventive medicine program.

Prevention by the Ounce

Preventive medicine is a young discipline, and youth—you'll be the first to agree—has its disadvantages!

In some cases, nutritional research has been long on zeal and short on method. Preliminary findings, issuing out of studies on rats and mice, often get reported as hard facts. On the other hand, intriguing findings are kept under wraps at times, lest rival investigators get wind of promising discoveries. And when lab research and population studies do identify a marker for disease prevention, it often is sensationalized or misrepresented to the public. Confusing? You bet.

The flurry surrounding the mineral selenium and the interest in fiber are two recent cases in point. Each *does* have a role to play in disease prevention, but the splashy headlines don't always reveal the full story. Selenium, for instance, is toxic at high levels. (The federal Food and Drug Administration [FDA] once banned selenium supplementation at high levels in animal feed because it caused blind staggering in field animals.) And yet many people take selenium supplements, believing that if a small amount has a protective effect, a larger amount will offer additional protection. That's patently untrue. You can bet the ranch on it. You need some selenium; in fact, some selenium in the diet may have a preventive effect against some cancers. Selenium is everywhere in food, however; deficiencies are virtually unknown in America. Megadose levels meanwhile are very dangerous.

Dietary fiber is another headline-maker, but you're probably still only partially informed. Only certain types of fiber help relieve constipation, for instance; only certain forms are helpful in reducing serum levels of cholesterol. And few people realize that fiber can bind minerals, making them unavailable to the body. How does this work? Fiber takes up minerals and "ushers" them right through the body, eliminating them with the stool. Some of these minerals, such as calcium, chromium and zinc, are especially important to the aging body. You shouldn't take a vitamin and mineral supplement with a bran cereal breakfast, for example, because the fiber will invalidate minerals. Remember, health faddism, while well-intentioned, can be as detrimental as healthful.

Another example? Many people over fifty take something called dolomite, a calcium and magnesium supplement. Few of them realize, however, that dolomite may also contain lead, arsenic, mercury and aluminum, which are dangerous in sufficient amounts. It's much smarter to get your calcium either from food, or from calcium gluconate or calcium carbonate supplements. (In fact, chewing on antacid tablets—those without sodium or aluminum—is the cheapest and easiest way to ensure calcium intake. More on that later!)

On the Palm Beach Diet, you'll receive what is, to the best of current knowledge, the optimal amounts of nutrients *for your age.* This book will help you make sense of all the diet and health information and advice you hear. You'll lose weight and manage—not damage—your health.

You may wonder why so little was known about the nutritional requirements of older people until now. And why has it taken until now to develop a diet for the middle-to-mature years? The answer is simple: Research on nutrition and aging has been limited, perhaps because until recently older people represented a much smaller segment of the population; little thought was given to the weight-loss problems of older Americans. Diet "gurus" aimed their recommendations at a younger audience, largely ignoring people over fifty.

Even the government has been in the dark as to what to recommend to people over fifty. Pick up a copy, for instance, of the National Research Council's Recommended Dietary Allowance—the government's suggestions for daily dietary vitamin and mineral intake. You'll find one set of vitamin and mineral requirements for adults twenty-three to fifty. You'll find another set of recommendations for those fifty-one-plus. The report doesn't tell you, however, that the Recommended Dietary Allowances for those over fifty are guesswork, based on studies conducted mainly with college volunteers. (Note, by the way, that the Recommended Dietary

Allowance differs somewhat from the Recommended Daily Allowance, or RDA, used on food and vitamin labeling. The Dietary Allowance is a standard *according to age;* the Daily Allowance [RDA] is, for the sake of convenience, a standard for nearly all persons over the age of four. For convenience, the vitamin recommendations of the Palm Beach Diet are quoted in terms of the Recommended Daily Allowance [RDA] used almost routinely throughout the food and vitamin industries. You'll find, however, that where I compare the Palm Beach Diet vitamin levels to those suggested by the government, I compare *Dietary* Allowances—those levels recommended for individuals fifty-one-plus years of age. Confusing? A bit. But don't worry: 5 mg. of vitamin B_6 is 5 mg., whatever you call it.)

Fortunately, times are changing. Research into nutrition and aging now is a hot ticket for government funding—understandably so. Given the rising life expectancy and recognizing that chronic illness is increasing in America, government and independent researchers are investigating ways to combat chronic disease with a real commitment. In 1974, the National Institute on Aging (NIA) was established to carry out biomedical and social research in the field of aging, for example. In conjunction with the U.S. Department of Agriculture, the NIA is overseeing work at the relatively new Human Nutrition Center at Tufts University in Boston. The center's mandate: Study how diet can delay or prevent the onset of degenerative conditions associated with the aging process. Part of that mandate is to help redefine the Recommended Daily Allowance of vitamins and minerals for those over fifty. In addition, a surge of university and independent research projects is discovering dietary links to a long and healthy life. Preventive medicine—like maturity—has finally come of age. This sunny fact has made the Palm Beach Diet, with its sound advice, the forerunner in its field.

Your Fat-Free Future

If a preventive medicine specialist like myself could help get you down to an ideal weight, what would that be? Sunken-cheeked skinny? Middle weight—the ideal weight range you read off insurance company weight charts? Or possibly, as you reach fifty and beyond, even a little over that?

The definition of "ideal weight" is controversial these days. For years, the medical community believed that to live a long life, and even to prolong life, the skinnier, the better—as long as the thin person was getting a full complement of nutrients. Recently, however, population studies seem to suggest that being on the plump side of those insurance weight tables is *not* a health threat.

In response to this evidence, the Metropolitan Life Insurance Company raised the ideal weight ranges on its latest weight tables. According to the 1983 Metropolitan Height and Weight Tables, ideal weights have been increased by 5 to 15 percent over previous recommendations! The desirable weight now for a woman with a medium-frame, at 5′4″, is set at 124–138 pounds. Incredible! The ideal weight range (at which the lowest mortality rate is assigned) for a 5′10″ man, medium-framed, now is 151–163 pounds.

These generous weight allowances have raised eyebrows—and excused some people from feeling they ought to diet. Why not resign yourself to being pleasingly—and according to these tables, "ideally"—plump?

Probably you've decided the main reason to diet is to *look* slim and trim. While I don't for a minute discount the value of the ego boost you get from looking attractive, I am more concerned with your health. I believe you should achieve and maintain a low weight because the data just described may be misleading. It may not be that the high-side of normal weight is healthy, but that being substantially *underweight* reduces life expectancy. Conditions associated with being too thin in advancing age—alcoholism, cigarette smoking and chronic illness—may well tilt the tables misleadingly.

In fact, fat doesn't score any health points. Many chronic conditions are caused or aggravated by substantial overweight. Ideal weight, when maintained on a diet that is rich in essential nutrients, promotes longevity.

Scientists have known for years that when animals are fed balanced low calorie diets, their lifespan is extended and their risk of developing later-life tumors is reduced! When rats are given calorie-restricted diets, for example, they live longer than those allowed to eat at will—up to 40 percent longer. Calorie restriction, in rats anyway, slows the rate at which diseases (including many cancers) emerge and progress. In one study, calorie restriction in mice slowed the decline in some aspects of the immune system, and delayed the appearance of autoimmune diseases.

What does the long life of a svelte mouse have to do with you and your diet? I am not advocating underweight as a way to prevent disease and prolong life—except perhaps for your rats! I am advocating ideal weight and a sound diet to protect you against disease and to help you live longer and better. Excess calories and poor nutrition are real threats to your health.

Some laboratory research suggests that substantial overweight may suppress the functioning of the immune system, for instance. One theory is that fats stored in the body interfere with the work of white blood cells. This is undesirable: White blood cells act like policemen on your body's "beat"—nosing out trouble-causing bacteria, viruses, irritants and cancer-causing agents. Like voracious computer-game characters, white blood cells gobble up foreign invaders. Obviously, they're vital to the efficiency of the immune system. If excess fat suppresses white blood cell activity, we can conclude that excess fat makes us less able to fight off illness.

Whatever the dynamic, obesity is a major risk factor in many chronic illnesses. Obesity increases the likelihood of heart disease, high blood pressure, uterine cancer, diabetes, gallbladder disease and gout. Overweight can increase the severity of arthritis, sleep disorders, varicose veins and hemorrhoids. Being fat seems to decrease resistance to infection, and may increase accident-proneness. It complicates surgery; it can adversely modify the quality of life. And it takes the pleasure out of physical activity.

Another point, too: Overweight makes some people doctor-shy—knowing full-well what the doctor will suggest. They're embarrassed to visit a doctor, and as a result a medical condition that may have been cured if caught early goes unattended, until it becomes chronic and debilitating.

Let's face it: Regardless of the increase in "ideal weight" tables, substantial overweight is a health hazard. Obesity—which is defined as 20 percent over ideal body weight—is a risk factor in many illnesses associated with aging. You needn't be sunken cheekbone-thin, but neither should you be satisfied to be pleasingly plump. *The weight that was ideal for you at twenty-five years old is the weight level you should strive for at fifty and beyond.* Your ideal weight can be roughly calculated this way: women should start at a figure of 100, and add five pounds for every inch they are over five feet tall. Example: A woman 5′4″ tall should weigh roughly 100 plus 20 (five pounds times four inches), or 120 pounds. Men start at a figure of 110, and likewise add five pounds for every inch they are over five feet tall. That figure is very roughly your ideal weight.

Old Fat vs. New Fat

There's another reason why I want you to strive to maintain the weight that was ideal for you during adulthood. Some interesting new research indicates that all fat may not be created equally. Creeping weight gain may be more health-hazardous than what doctors call "uncomplicated" obesity—substantial overweight since childhood that remains relatively stable during the adult years.

What's the difference between "old" fat and "new" fat? There are biomedical differences. The marker of lifetime overweight generally is a large *number* of fat cells. A marker of weight-gain later in life is the increased *size* of existing fat cells. The difference doesn't end there: The relationship of those two different kinds of fat to health may be different, too.

One study, for example, found that weight gain after the age of twenty was more closely related to the incidence of stroke than was weight per se at age twenty. It may be that weight gain after this age can be particularly hazardous; studies indicate it may be a factor contributing to stroke and hardening of the arteries. Most of these studies are preliminary and most bear repeating. More work is under way now.

What this means to you: Yo-yo dieting—in which weight fluctuates between highs and lows—may be more health-damaging than we thought. It means that diets which let you "eat all you want" of certain fatty foods or allow you to binge at prescribed intervals may invite health problems. Don't risk your health! If you have been gaining weight since age twenty, as many people have, you need to lose weight—but smartly and permanently.

CHAPTER 3

America's Aged Elite—and Your Elite Body

The median age in Palm Beach is fifty-eight. And when a local newspaper recently polled its readers, three-quarters of the respondents claimed an income of $50,000 or more—or wouldn't tell. But this isn't what sociologists mean by America's aged elite. More Americans are living longer, and debunking the image of a washed-up old age. This select group—pioneers in "maturity management"—remains vigorous, interested, sparkling. Against the statistical odds, they're bucking old-age illness; they're entering their later years with optimism and with their eyes wide open. Who are they? How do they live?

There are a number of clues that older Americans are increasingly astute all around. Between 1960 and 1980, for instance, the number of older persons with four years of high school or more doubled. Older Americans today also are financially better off than ever before: The median income of those over sixty-five has risen in recent years faster than income levels for the overall population.

These sorts of facts tilt at preconceived notions of grandma and grandpa shuffling around the house, puzzled by the modern world and uncertain how to act within it. Today's elderly and soon-to-be elderly have high expectations, plenty of chutzpah. There are some other heartening tip-offs that times are changing:

• A significant number of older persons tested for intellectual performance at a university in California showed an improvement with age. Even between the ages of seventy-four and eighty-one, almost 10 percent of people tested performed better than they had at younger ages. This belies the belief that intelligence necessarily falls away during the later years. Middle-aged people whose lifestyles and attitudes are flexible are most likely to maintain their intellectual abilities later in life.

• The "young" old are the heaviest voters in national elections. The fifty-five to sixty-four age group has the highest participation rate while the sixty-five to seventy-four age group is next highest.

• Two-thirds of all homes owned free and clear are maintained by an older person.

• Only 5 percent of people aged sixty-five or older live in nursing homes.

• Retirement may not be the emotional and health crisis it's been made out to be. A three-year study in Boston indicated that the physical health of 260 men who had retired was no different than the health of 500 of their still-working peers.

That's America's aged elite for you. Still realizing their potential. Involved in the world. Shaping their lives for the better. And yet, if there's one area in which many otherwise savvy over-fifties slip up, it's the area of health and well-being. A good chunk of the millions of Americans who are overweight are fifty or older. Many of them are candidates for weight-related health problems that could be avoided. Why aren't they coping successfully in this area of their lives, too?

Blame ignorance and fear, for the most part. Thank goodness that ignorance and fear can be dispelled. Trust me on this: Fear is much more intimidating than knowledge.

Might you, for instance, secretly fear being thinner? Are you just a little bit afraid of being more attractive? Think hard on this one. You may be hiding behind that fat. You may fear change—even though you're dissatisfied with your chubby status quo! *Try not to fear change. Let change happen. You'll be happier for it.*

Do you have a mental block against anything and everything medical? Do you fear seeing a doctor? Do you treat your body as a stranger and regard aging as a calamitous assault on your well-being? Don't! I'll tell you why: Fear makes you especially vulnerable to misinformation and quackery. When you refuse to confront your diet and health concerns directly, you will likely deal with them indirectly—by taking a friend's questionable advice or acting upon half-truths you read and hear, for example.

I find it amazing that in the last few years, for instance, you've been told that you can safeguard your health and even reverse existing illness through megavitamin therapy alone. There's much more to health through nutrition than a vitamin pill. Other diet and nutrition advice has been even tougher to track. Starch-blockers were supposed to help you lose weight without dieting—and then starch-blockers were banned. "Magic" enzymes could melt fat; magic enzymes were debunked. Vitamin E could improve your sex life, and then the edict came down: Fat chance. Low-carbohydrate diets were greeted like tablets from the mountain, but then the low-carbohydrate diets proved to work only temporarily, and were shown to have dangerous side effects. My point is that even the most astute among you, in a desperate desire to lose weight and stay healthy, may have been duped by misinformation and outright quackery.

I want you to understand just how fantastic and elite a machine the human body is. You don't have to fear it; you can take tremendous pride in it. Need convincing? Here's some supporting evidence:

- Most of the body's functions are carried out automatically: You don't have to think about them! Your body automatically digests food. It knows how to keep your temperature at 98.6° F in a hot climate or in a cold room. It makes you rest when necessary. It carries thoughts faster than any computer can.

- Your heart will beat over three billion times by the age of eighty, and continue for another decade or two if you take care of it.

- You could live without your gallbladder, appendix and tonsils. You need only one kidney and about half of your liver!

- When you catch cold, it's not medication that cures it. If you should break a leg, it's not the cast that mends the break. It's not drugs or casts or bandages that heal us. Healing comes from within the body. The natural tendency is toward healing. This recuperative power not only heals, but helps resist disease as well.

Your Fifty-Plus Body—a Cook's Tour

You look in the mirror now, and you look a bit different than you did at thirty or forty. You call it age. And time can alter your looks, no denying it. And yet, too often, what we take as signs of aging are really signs of poor nutrition.

I can hear you now. "Poor nutrition!" you laugh. "*Over*abundance is my problem." But wait. What are you getting in your meals and snacks? Do you realize that your nutritional needs are changing, now that you're fifty or more? That, now, even a seemingly healthy diet can accelerate the aging process? Let me explain.

You need fewer calories now, for example. The rate at which your body works decreases with age. This metabolic rate can decrease by about 20 percent between the ages of twenty and ninety. The amount of food you eat really counts now.

At the same time, you need more of some vitamins and minerals than you once did. *With age, your ability to absorb and to use certain nutrients decreases.* The absorptive cells of the intestines, for instance, lose some efficiency in taking nutrients from food. The lining of the small intestine becomes thinner, with fewer absorptive cells, and fewer blood vessels to carry nutrients to other parts of the body. Stomach acid that is important to absorption decreases. These changes affect certain vitamins and minerals more than it does others: Iron and vitamin B_{12} appear especially vulnerable to the decreased-absorption dynamic of aging.

Your body's ability to use minerals can also take a tumble. Calcium, for instance, is used less efficiently beginning at about the age of forty. Once more, some people tend to eat fewer calcium-rich foods (such as milk, cheese, ice cream) as they get older. This double-whammy—less calcium, less readily used—puts many people over fifty at risk of calcium depletion.

In designing the Palm Beach Diet we have paid close attention to this problem. *Once you reach fifty or more, an adequate diet no longer guarantees adequate nutrition.* Your daily requirement of certain vitamins and minerals may be higher than you suspect, in order to achieve adequate *body* levels of these nutrients. You have to get more, in other words, in order to get enough! I'll outline specifically what those needs are in Chapter 4.

In addition, after you pass fifty, your body doesn't use some nutrients as efficiently once they are absorbed. So we need to compensate again. For example, early findings suggest that aging cells take up nutrients less readily than do younger cells: In one laboratory experiment, zinc absorption by aged lung cells was 40 percent lower than in young lung cells. Now that you're older, you may require higher levels of some nutrients, either to absorb or use sufficient amounts.

Your protein needs, now that you're fifty or more, may be changing as well. Research at the Massachusetts Institute of Technology concluded that the mature individual may have an increased protein requirement. This finding, however, like many in the field of nutrition, is controversial: Other work indicates that protein need doesn't change with age. Once more, isolated findings of this sort must be given a long look. A high protein diet carries certain *disadvantages* for those fifty-plus, as I'll explain later on. Based on this knowledge, the Palm Beach Diet strikes an optimal protein balance for those fifty or more. I should mention here that people who are big meat-eaters probably get far too much protein anyway. Remember protein also comes in fish, poultry, eggs, cheese, milk, nuts, breads, cereals, and beans, as well as in meat. The typical American diet contains more protein than is necessary.

What about other physical changes that occur with age? Many affect the way in which you metabolize and utilize nutrients and the way in which your body responds to the chemistry of food. Because it is scientifically based, the Palm Beach Diet responds to these changes, adjusting food chemistry to accommodate the biological shifts of aging. For example:

• As you grow older, you produce less gastric acid and fewer digestive enzymes in the stomach. (While you may *feel* you have a more acid stomach than you once did, there actually is less acid in the stomach as you grow older. That acidic feeling is probably gas.) This decreased production interferes with iron absorption, for example. Low body levels of iron, in turn, can cause anemia. How much of these digestive substances you lose with age varies considerably: Some of us maintain youthful amounts, while others produce almost no gastric acid, for instance, in later life. On the Palm Beach Diet, you'll get plenty of iron for a number of reasons, including this fact of lowered digestive potential.

• Another physical age-change is a reduction in the secretion of digestive juices by the gallbladder, the pancreas and the small intestine. While it is not a big problem, this loss inhibits your ability to digest fat and may cause gas. This is one of several reasons why the Palm Beach Diet is low in fat.

• With age, the kidneys become a little less efficient at elimination. Plenty of liquids in the diet can compensate by diluting the urine. You'll find a generous liquid allowance on the Palm Beach Diet—although people who have heart failure or liver disease should check with their doctor before undertaking a high-liquid diet. Exercise is another way to keep kidneys working at their best, by boosting circulation. The Palm Beach Diet, remember, advocates exercise as an essential part of your new lifestyle.

• Moving down the digestive "trail," another marker of maturity is the very common problem of constipation and the development of pouches in the wall of the intestine called *diverticuli.* In the United States, about half of us can expect to develop these pesky diverticuli by the age of seventy! Both constipation and diverticulosis can be prevented by a diet that contains plenty of fiber. Fiber is a crucial ingredient in any diet directed at people over fifty. In this case, however, fiber doesn't mean gluey roughage or barrels of beans. Beans can cause gas. On the Palm Beach Diet, your fiber will come from more enticing foods.

> **Palm Beach Postscript:** It's important to know that some forms of irritable bowel and colitis can actually be aggravated by a high-fiber diet. If you have either condition, the Palm Beach Diet is *not* for you. Both conditions are easily diagnosed by a doctor, should you have any doubts.

• Heartburn is a common complaint among people who are older and overweight. Something called *gastroesophageal reflux* is often to blame. What happens? Acid rushes back up into the esophagus from the stomach; this usually is due to a "loose" valve that allows acid and stomach contents to bubble back up into the esophagus. The most bothersome and most common result is heartburn. Your diet can be of some help in avoiding this syndrome; such substances as fat, chocolate, alcohol, peppermint, cigarettes and certain drugs can aggravate gas and heartburn by loosening up the valve. The Palm Beach Diet can't solve this problem, but it will not aggravate it as much as some other diets.

These are the sorts of physical changes that occur in all of us over time. Most are not health threats; at worst, many are mere nuisances.

You can help ensure that these physical changes don't become health worries. Diet is your vehicle. While a preventive diet can't *guarantee* you'll never have a health problem, it can, in many cases, mean the difference between health and illness. On the Palm Beach

Diet—the ultimate preventive plan—you protect your health while you lose weight. You also protect your health with exercise. How's that for being astute?

Now let's turn to the nitty-gritty "ingredients" of the diet itself—nutrients that can make you look and feel years younger.

> **Palm Beach Postscript:** The Palm Beach Diet addresses the progressive digestive changes with age in healthy individuals. It cannot cure disease; anyone who is being treated for disease of the digestive tract may already have been prescribed a special diet by their doctor. While the Palm Beach Diet may be compatible with your prescribed diet, check with your doctor before starting this or any other diet. Remember not to go off any medication you may be taking.

CHAPTER 4

Palm Beach Health Dividends—Vitamins and Minerals

Do people resemble elephants? Hardly. Where then do otherwise sensible people get the notion that their health depends on taking mammoth amounts of vitamins and minerals?

Don't get me wrong. I'm not some sort of antivitamin vigilante. In fact, the Palm Beach Diet supplies more than the standard recommendation of many vitamins and minerals. I want to make you a believer in the value of vitamins and minerals, but you don't need a *vat* of vitamin supplements to stay healthy.

Let's look, for instance, at the largest mineral dosage you'll receive on this diet. You'll be getting about 1000–1200 milligrams (mg.) of calcium each day. That amount of calcium can be supplied in a tablet the size of a typical baby aspirin! Many of the other minerals you'll receive every day are measured in micrograms (mcg.), or one-millionth of a gram. Important as minerals are, your daily need for most minerals is so small, each dosage could dance on the point of a straight pin. *My point:*

Let's put the vogue for vitamins and minerals in perspective. What you want—and what this diet delivers to you—is the optimal amount of each nutrient.

Alas, identifying the perfect nutritional balance for people over fifty isn't easy. It's a little like trying to balance a checkbook when you've a *vague* idea of your assets and only a *fuzzy* notion of how many checks you wrote for what amount. We know your body is changing with age, for example; we can adjust nutrient recommendations to compensate for many of these natural changes. We know which vitamins and minerals the older American is likely to be "low" on. This is very helpful. What's confounding, though, are the field and laboratory studies of nutritional needs—findings don't always agree. Different "accounting" methods of determining vitamin and mineral levels for older individuals can yield different results.

An example: Investigators asked older people to list what they had eaten over the past week and then analyzed their menus; in many cases, they found inadequate sources of certain vitamins and minerals—especially calcium, iron, vitamin A, vitamin B_1 and folic acid. Yet when another group of researchers examined blood levels of nutrients in a different group of older individuals, the "low" items were protein and vitamins A and C. Meanwhile, in the face of all these controversial and conflicting reports, you're drumming your fingers on the dining room table, wondering whether to skip the eggs, eat more carrots or perhaps develop a taste for soybeans! It's exasperating all around.

My philosophy is straightforward. I've looked at the evidence. I've consulted the experts. Where there is controversy or uncertainty, I tell you so; then I choose what my experience tells me is most helpful and yet safe. There is all you need to know about these important little nutrients in the following pages.

The Palm Beach Nutrient Honor Roll

Certain vitamins and minerals are especially important to the fifty-plus system. Charted here are the key vitamins and minerals of the Palm Beach Diet. They're not the only nutrients you'll receive, but these are the ones that deserve special attention.

THE PALM BEACH DIET'S VITAMIN AND MINERAL PORTFOLIO

	The U.S. Recommended Dietary Allowance is:		The Palm Beach Diet contains:
	Men 51 +	Women 51 +	
Vitamin A	5000 I.U.	4000 I.U.	5000–10,000 I.U.
Vitamin B_1	1.2 mg.	1 mg.	1.2–2 mg.
Vitamin B_6	2.2 mg.	2 mg.	5–10 mg.
Vitamin B_{12}	3 mcg.	3 mcg.	3–6 mcg.
Folic acid	400 mcg.	400 mcg.	400 mcg.
Vitamin C	60 mg.	60 mg.	200 mg.
Vitamin D	200 I.U.	200 I.U.	400 I.U.
Vitamin E	15 I.U.	12 I.U.	50–100 I.U.
Iron	10 mg.	10 mg.	20–30 mg.
Zinc	15 mg.	15 mg.	20–25 mg.
Calcium	800 mg.	800 mg.	1000–1200 mg.

The chart compares the key nutrients you receive on the diet with the Recommended Dietary Allowances set by the federal government. In each case, you receive more than the standard recommended amount, but not an unsafe excessive amount. The exception is folic acid: While folic acid tends to be low in the diet of many older Americans, too much folic acid may mask a deficiency of vitamin B_{12}, which could be health-endangering. On the Palm Beach Diet, you'll get the Recommended Dietary Allowance of folic acid, set at 400 micrograms each day.

Incidentally, the attribution "I.U." as used here stands for International Units, a complex measure of the ability of a vitamin to promote growth or cure deficiency. Vitamins A, D and E frequently are referred to in terms of International Units.

Vitamin A

The U.S. Recommended Dietary Allowance for individuals 51-plus is:	The Palm Beach Diet contains:
5000 I.U. for men 4000 I.U. for women	5000–10,000 I.U.

Abundant in: carrots, liver, margarine, butter, milk, cheese, dark yellow/orange fruits and vegetables

Vitamin A may lower susceptibility to certain forms of cancer, according to the 1982 report from the National Academy of Science entitled *Diet, Nutrition and Cancer.* Vitamin A also maintains ability to fight infection, keeps skin normal and helps keep eyes healthy and able to see at night.

The case for getting enough vitamin A is strong—although not without controversy. A recent investigation suggests that it may be something *else* in vitamin A-high vegetables that exerts a protective effect against some cancers, and not necessarily vitamin A itself. This possibility only confirms my belief that it's much healthier to get your vitamins and minerals from food, and not strictly from a vitamin bottle.

Vitamin A is tricky, however, because it is toxic in large doses. It is foolhardy to take megadose supplements of vitamin A. The smart way to get vitamin A is in your diet. The body converts something called carotene in dark green and yellow/orange vegetables and fruits *into* vitamin A, but it only converts what it needs, so there is no danger of overdose. Clever body! And, now, clever you!

Carotene-rich foods such as carrots, broccoli, parsley, spinach, asparagus and sweet potatoes are abundant on the Palm Beach Diet. The Palm Beach Diet's 5,000–10,000 I.U. of vitamin A is generally held as a safe level. At the same time, it more than ensures against vitamin A deficiency linked with susceptibility to certain forms of tumors.

Vitamin B_1 (Thiamine)

The U.S. Recommended Dietary Allowance for individuals 51-plus is:	The Palm Beach Diet contains:
1.2 mg. for men 1.0 mg. for women	1.2–2 mg.

Abundant in: whole grains, green vegetables, raisins, pork, organ meats, peanuts, wheat germ, milk, dried beans, peas

The case isn't nailed shut, but it looks as if we need more of certain B vitamins as we grow older. Four of the "Bs" are of special concern. Thiamine, or vitamin B_1, is frequently found to be marginally deficient in older Americans. That's *one* red flag. Vitamin B_1 is important to the mature system. Too little of it, and fatigue and aloofness can set in—and even be mistaken for mental deterioration. The Palm Beach Diet delivers roughly twice the RDA of vitamin B_1.

Before I suggest what vitamin B_6 will do perhaps I should tell you what it *won't* do. Just about everything you read about B_6 in the popular press these days is mistaken.

First is the recent and popular notion that vitamin B_6 relieves water retention (edema). Some doctors prescribe megadoses of B_6 for premenstrual edema. However, as stated uncategorically in a recent *Harvard Medical School Health Letter:* "No responsible investigator has reported a study showing that high doses are effective in reducing edema."

Vitamin B_6 (Pyridoxine)

The U.S. Recommended Dietary Allowance for individuals 51-plus is:	The Palm Beach Diet contains:
2.2 mg. for men 2.0 mg. for women	5–10 mg.

Abundant in: wheat germ, lean meat, organ meats, milk, whole grains, beans

Vitamin B_6 also has been touted as having a protective effect against some diseases of the arteries. The theory is that B_6 may prevent the amino acid methionine (a protein component especially abundant in meats) from being converted in the body to a toxic chemical that wreaks havoc with the arteries. That conclusion is based on animal studies—and simply hasn't been duplicated satisfactorily. There is no point in taking B_6 to prevent hardening of the arteries.

Until recently vitamin B_6 was thought to be nontoxic; however, recent reports indicate that vitamin B_6 can cause severe side effects at megadose levels. A report in *The New England Journal of Medicine* reveals that seven adults taking megadoses of B_6 developed such symptoms as unsteadiness in walking, clumsiness and loss of sensation in the hands and feet. A deterioration of nerve fibers may be to blame—a severe side effect indeed. The levels cited were very high: 200 mg. to 6 g. per day, many times greater than the amount on the Palm Beach Diet.

The Palm Beach Diet is rich in vitamin B_6 foods, but far short of overdose levels. You receive enough of the vitamin for the body to do its B_6 "thing"—that is, make amino acids, fatty acids, hemoglobin and other biochemical necessities.

Vitamin B_{12}

The U.S. Recommended Dietary Allowance for individuals 51-plus is:	The Palm Beach Diet contains:
3 mcg. for men 3 mcg. for women	3–6 mcg.

Abundant in: meat, milk and other dairy products, poultry, fish

Vitamin B_{12} is another sticky wicket. If there's one vitamin associated with aging, it's vitamin B_{12}. It's common practice to give older people a "booster injection" of B_{12}: Certain anemic conditions in older individuals are thought to benefit from B_{12} injections—one justifiably, as I'll explain later. Most often, though, B_{12} injections, while not harmful, help very few people.

In fact, the evidence shows clearly that most elderly persons are not deficient in vitamin B_{12}. One study found no B_{12} deficiency among subjects aged sixty to eighty-seven. Marginal deficiency of vitamin B_{12}, in fact, doesn't appear to be as prevalent as deficiencies of other vitamins. (When vitamin B_{12} deficiency does occur, it generally is in vegetarians or in those people with pernicious anemia, certain stomach or rare metabolic conditions, or certain diseases of the small bowel.)

The three to six daily micrograms of vitamin B_{12} on the Palm Beach Diet is up to double the Recommended Dietary Allowance. That amount will compensate in most cases for normal decline in nutrient absorption associated with aging. Vitamin B_{12}, though, is a special case, in that absorption by the body depends on what's called an "intrinsic factor"— something found in the stomach's secretions—to take the B_{12} across the wall of the small intestine and into the bloodstream. With age, most people produce a little less of this substance; a few older people produce too little of it. Some people with pernicious anemia do not absorb vitamin B_{12} at all because they do not have intrinsic factor. They may require B_{12} injections. However, very few of us have to worry about being short on intrinsic factor. In fact, almost everyone who eats red meat twice a week has roughly a three-to-five-year supply of B_{12} in the liver.

Folic Acid

The U.S. Recommended Dietary Allowance for individuals 51-plus is:	The Palm Beach Diet contains:
400 mcg. for men 400 mcg. for women	400 mcg.

Abundant in: liver, green and leafy vegetables, beans, peas

Two separate studies found almost 60 percent of elderly persons to be at risk of folic acid deficiency. If your diet is low in folate-high foods, you are especially vulnerable. On the Palm Beach Diet, you get the Recommended Dietary Allowance of folic acid. I consider it a key nutrient because (*a*) deficiency is common; (*b*) it's essential in the prevention of anemia; and (*c*) even a mild deficiency has been linked with inflammation of the gums.

That isn't an invitation, though, to take *more* folic acid. In fact, high doses can pull a punch on the system and mask vitamin B_{12} deficiency. Because of this danger the amount of folic acid you can buy without a prescription is limited by law.

A special note on B vitamins and the brain: Even subtle deficiencies of B vitamins like niacin can cause what's called "false senility" in the elderly. The brain is the first organ to suffer when B vitamins run low because the brain needs the Bs to metabolize glucose for energy. Without them, there's a slowdown of mental functioning, and possible confusion resembling senility. The Palm Beach Diet assures against deficiency.

Vitamin C

The U.S. Recommended Dietary Allowance for individuals 51-plus is:	The Palm Beach Diet contains:
60 mg. for men 60 mg. for women	200 mg.

Abundant in: citrus fruits, tomatoes, cantaloupe, strawberries, broccoli, cabbage, peppers, potatoes

We can put a man on the moon and a five-year-old at a computer terminal, but we still can't determine exactly what vitamin C can and cannot do in the body. Some brave new world!

We do know this much: Vitamin C appears to help protect us against pollutants and poisons; it helps increase resistance to infection; it prevents the conversion of nitrates found in foods into nitrosamines—substances known to cause cancer. It also protects vitamins A and E from degradation by other substances. It aids in iron absorption, speeds healing of wounds and strengthens blood vessels. And there's still more.

Vitamin C may play a role in the reduction of what is intriguingly called "free radical activity." Free radicals are very reactive compounds which bind to cells in the body, interfering with their activity. Free radicals have been implicated in the aging process and in certain diseases. Vitamin C may help curb these rascal compounds.

Vitamin C also may reduce the symptoms of a common cold by about one-third. (But it can't prevent the *onset* of a cold, no matter what you've heard!) Vitamin C in substantial amounts also appears to arrest plaque formation on the teeth and gums. Plaque is gummy deposits of bacteria which erode teeth and contribute to gum disease.

All of which makes "C" sound like a miracle vitamin. It *is* a most versatile nutrient, but even vitamin C—everyone's favorite vitamin supplement—shouldn't be taken in elephant doses of a gram or more. It's simply not true that if a moderate amount is helpful, a large amount will be *more* helpful.

Some warnings: Megadoses of vitamin C can cause nausea, abdominal cramps and diarrhea. Chronic overuse can result in kidney stones. Too much of this good thing can do exactly the opposite of what you take it for—that is, *reduce* the ability of the immune system to fight infection.

Megadoses also are wasteful. Megadoses of vitamin C don't get used efficiently by the body: The body uses what vitamin C it needs and excretes the rest. One study found that from a daily intake of 180 mg. of vitamin C, 60 percent was excreted in the urine. At a monster level of 2 g. (2000 mg.) of vitamin C per day, a whopping 90 percent was flushed out with urine.

The Palm Beach Diet provides, on average, 200 mg. of vitamin C per day. That's more than enough to ensure your receiving its important benefits, without overdoing.

Vitamin D

The U.S. Recommended Dietary Allowance for individuals 51-plus is:	The Palm Beach Diet contains:
200 I.U. for men 200 I.U. for women	400 I.U.

Abundant in: fish, eggs, chicken liver, milk

Here's another instance in which you walk a biochemical tightrope between deficiency and overdose.

Vitamin D is important for a big reason: Without it, calcium cannot be absorbed by the body. Too little vitamin D depresses calcium "uptake," which can result in soft bones. On the other hand, too much vitamin D increases calcium absorption, possibly promotes hardening of the arteries, and can cause calcium deposits such as kidney stones. If you guess that you want to avoid both syndromes, you've guessed right.

The Palm Beach Diet provides about 400 I.U. of vitamin D per day in your food and in your multivitamin supplement combined. That's moderately more than the Recommended Dietary Allowance, but well within safety limits.

Your vitamin D levels are greatly affected, too, by the amount of sun exposure you get. You can meet all of your vitamin D requirement by spending substantial time outdoors in sunlight. Even ten minutes of exposure every other day boosts body levels of vitamin D—although it won't, by itself, satisfy your full need. (Of course, ten minutes in Palm Beach is more vitamin D-productive than ten minutes in Montreal, where the sunlight is less intense!)

Where does this leave you and vitamin D? Guessing, a bit. While the vitamin D recommendation on the Palm Beach Diet ideally is 400 I.U. per day, your body levels of "D" will depend on how often you're outdoors, how intense the sun is, whether or not you use milk on the diet with coffee or tea, and the vitamin D contents of the multivitamin/mineral supplement you choose. Confusing? A little, but don't worry—given that vitamin D is stored in the body (you've got some in reserve) *and* that you're getting more on the diet, you can rest easy that your vitamin D level is about right.

Vitamin E figures closely in the aging process. One "hat" it wears, for instance, is labeled *antioxidant.*

Vitamin E

The U.S. Recommended Dietary Allowance for individuals 51-plus is:	The Palm Beach Diet contains:
15 I.U. for men 12 I.U. for women	50–100 I.U.

Abundant in: vegetable oil, margarine, nuts, wheat germ

An antioxidant is a substance which can prevent an unwanted chemical reaction or two in the body. Remember meeting "free radicals" a few pages back? Free radicals are molecule fragments caused when oxygen changes the structure of, say, polyunsaturated fats.

Free radicals are biochemical bad guys. They do just what you might expect unchecked hell-raisers to do: They hot-rod among body cells, causing damage. They may even form rigid bridges between cells, a process called *biomolecular crosslinking.* This is more potentially bad news. Some researchers have hypothesized that this chain reaction, kicked off by the mix of fats and oxygen, can cause cancer. It also may encourage such age-associated events as cellular debilitation, wrinkling and accelerated formation of pigments and age spots thought to "clog" aging cells. The theory then comes full circle: Vitamin E, because it can prevent oxygen from altering the chemical structure of fats, may, by extension, help prevent cancer.

Free radical theory now is a "hot" area of research. Current findings, though, are slightly frustrating. At one university, for example, very large doses of vitamin E are being given to colon cancer patients. Yet the investigators aren't certain that the vitamin is even going to the cells in the colon! It's a case, it seems, where theory and laboratory experiments are tidy—but just try to put theory into practice with people!

Scientists have found that when they combine free radical molecules with vitamin E molecules, the vitamin E prevents free radicals (those rascals!) from combining with oxygen. It's not that straightforward in the human body, though; there's no guarantee that the vitamin will be taken up by free radical-damaged, or free radical-vulnerable, cells. And a human may not be able to absorb enough vitamin E to make a difference. (In order to achieve the same 1:1 vitamin E/free radical ratio you can achieve in a test tube, you'd have to consume a washtub of vitamin E. And you wouldn't absorb it all.) The point: No one has yet shown that vitamin E even gets to the places it's supposed to go, or in sufficient quantities to do any good. Everyone wants the free radical-vitamin E theory to be true . . . but we can't yet say so with any certainty.

Meanwhile, for the purposes of the Palm Beach Diet, my summation is that if you don't have adequate quantities of vitamin E, you may be producing an environment in which free radicals can be produced. No one knows for sure, remember.

> **Palm Beach Postscript:** Do not interpret the preceding to read that vitamin E can *cure* cancer. It cannot. No vitamin should be taken as replacement therapy for traditional methods of treatment.

Vitamin E also can alleviate some cases of a condition called *intermittent claudication.* You know it as leg cramp—often severe pain in the muscles of the legs and feet caused by the obstruction of blood flow. Levels of at least 400 I.U. of vitamin E alleviate the spasms and cramping in some cases. Don't ask why: Vitamin E's effect on leg cramps remains a mystery.

Iron

The U.S. Recommended Dietary Allowance for individuals 51-plus is:	The Palm Beach Diet contains:
10 mg. for men 10 mg. for women	20–30 mg.
(18 mg. for women under 51)	

Abundant in: red meat, liver, enriched bread, oysters, clams, raisins, beans

When we say someone looks anemic, we generally mean he or she looks pale. Anemia, however, is a more serious condition than mere complexion "wash-out"—especially if you're fifty or more. It means that your red blood-cell count is low; this can result in shortness of breath and rapid heart rhythm. Headaches and loss of concentration also may signal anemia. In severe cases, reduction of oxygen delivered by the bloodstream to the brain can result in impaired brain function. Iron deficiency *causes* anemia.

Taking too much iron, on the other hand, can cause iron *overloading:* Iron must be taken within a cautious dosage range. And just to thicken the plot even more: Age affects the way the body absorbs iron. In some, the ability to absorb iron decreases with age: At fifty or more, you may need a little more iron in order to get enough.

To cover your needs, then, the Palm Beach Diet provides 20–30 mg./day of iron. This should be enough to meet or exceed the Recommended Dietary Allowance, even in cases of decreased absorption, or iron loss due to microscopic gastrointestinal bleeding. This amount is not high enough to risk overdose symptoms, however.

Believe it or not, 20–30 mg. of iron is hard to come by, even in a carefully balanced diet. Iron doesn't grow on trees! (Well, that's not completely true: Iron is contained in some vegetables, fruits and nuts, but plant-source iron isn't absorbed as well as iron from red meat.) For this reason, you're asked to take a multivitamin/mineral supplement containing iron while you diet. The supplement should contain about 10 mg. of iron—enough to fortify the iron content of your meals.

By the way, you also "up" your iron quota every morning of the Palm Beach Diet. You do so by taking your multivitamin/mineral supplement with fruit: Most fruit contains vitamin C which helps the body absorb iron.

> **Palm Beach Postscript:** A few individuals may be at risk of iron overload. If you have anemia which is not due to iron deficiency, or cirrhosis, Parkinsonism, diabetes, or have been taking iron supplements for several years, check with your doctor before supplementing your diet with iron. This is especially good advice for men, who do not lose iron over a lifetime from menstrual bleeding, and therefore are more likely to retain high body levels of iron. Too much iron in the diet can cause iron deposits in the liver, pancreas, heart and the skin, and can be particularly dangerous. Symptoms of iron overload usually manifest themselves after the age of forty, and include a bronze cast to the skin and, often, depression.

Zinc

The U.S. Recommended Dietary Allowance for individuals 51-plus is:	The Palm Beach Diet contains:
15 mg. for men 15 mg. for women	20–25 mg.

Abundant in: meat, poultry, fish, milk, eggs

Zinc sounds about as enticing as root-canal work, but don't shrug it off as a dietary clunker. Zinc's role in aging—or, more exactly, in the symptoms of aging—is a starring role.

What are investigators discovering about zinc? It's vital to the workings of the immune system, which helps you fight disease. It's a prime mover in wound healing, for instance. Zinc also can "recharge"senses of taste and smell that have been dulled by zinc deficiency. (This doesn't mean zinc can make you a wine connoisseur, mind you, if you can't now tell the difference between Chardonnay and Côtes du Rhone! It *can* improve your sensation of taste, however, which makes your food taste more appealing, if you've been low on zinc all along.)

Zinc shares a couple of traits with iron. Both minerals are better absorbed from animal and fish sources than from plant sources. Once more, zinc needs, like iron needs, can be greatly affected by illnesses which can afflict mature individuals, including kidney failure and cirrhosis.

Getting enough zinc can be a little tricky. A substance found in grains and vegetables, called *phytic acid,* can be a real obstacle, grabbing up zinc and moving it right through the system without being absorbed. For this reason, the Palm Beach Diet generally separates zinc-high foods from fiber-high foods.

That's the good news about zinc. The qualifying news is that high levels of zinc to *copper* in the body can pull a tricky chemical punch—decreasing the amount of heart-protective HDL cholesterol substantially. HDL cholesterol is a "good guy" cholesterol because it protects against heart disease—one convincing reason not to megadose zinc. Excessive zinc also causes well-established side effects, such as abdominal pain, anemia, nausea and fever. Zinc overloading also may cause elevated cholesterol levels. Balance—optimal balance—is key again. You don't want too much or too little zinc. The

Palm Beach Diet's 20–25 mg./day establishes an appropriate range for people over fifty.

Chromium

Abundant in: whole grains, seafood, cheese, fresh fruits and vegetables.

There is not a U.S. Recommended Dietary Allowance for this trace mineral. Instead, you get an "estimated safe and adequate daily intake" of 50–200 mcg. (that's *micrograms*)—very little indeed. The Palm Beach plan more than meets this chromium level, for two reasons: *One:* Several reports tell us that body levels of chromium decrease with age; *Two:* Chromium's big job in the body is aiding in sugar metabolism. Sugar metabolism becomes impaired in many older people, and sufficient chromium in the diet is important.

Want specifics? Here's one finding, among a group of elderly people. Half of the group was found to have an impaired ability to digest sugars—meaning they either exhibited some symptoms of diabetes, or they actually had diabetes. When given supplementary chromium, however, all subjects handled sugar normally.

This isn't license, though, to jump to conclusions—and land on the nearest bottle of chromium pills. Chromium supplements are not necessary on this, or almost any sound, diet. And as possible effects of chromium overdose are not known, I don't recommend chromium supplements. The Palm Beach Diet is rich in chromium-high foods, so just enjoy what you take in naturally.

Palm Beach Postscript: Chromium supplementation should *never* be used as replacement therapy for insulin in the case of diabetes. It will not work.

Selenium

Abundant in: seafood, asparagus, garlic, mushrooms, whole wheat

Selenium is another trace mineral given an "estimated safe and adequate daily intake" notation by the federal government. Like chromium, that level is set at a scant 50–200 mcg./day. The Palm Beach Diet is a seafood bonanza, so you needn't worry that you won't get enough of this "hot" nutrient while you're dieting.

Why is there a stir about selenium? It appears to act in the body with vitamin E. Like "E," selenium is an antioxidant—it counteracts oxygen's potentially harmful effects on body fats. According to the National Academy of Science's report *Diet, Nutrition and Cancer,* adequate-to-high selenium intake has been correlated with a decreased risk of certain cancers, although the report declines from drawing any firm conclusions on the basis of the present limited evidence.

So the Palm Beach Diet supplies you with foods rich in selenium, but discourages supplementation. Recently, a fifty-seven-year-old woman went bald after mistakenly taking huge amounts of selenium supplements over a two-month period!

The selenium content of plant foods is difficult to measure, incidentally. It depends on the selenium content of the soil in which they're grown, but rest easy: A selenium deficiency has *never* been reported in the United States except in people who are being fed intravenously on a long-term basis.

Palm Beach Postscript: Both selenium and chromium in excess may be harmful.

CHAPTER 5

Palm Beach Health Dividends—Biochemical Balances

Vitamins and minerals, you already know about. You see and read reports on the "wonders" of this vitamin or that mineral. On top of this hoopla, well-meaning family members and friends may suggest you try this or that nutrient to alleviate or cure a particular health complaint. Even if much of the information funneled your way is wrong, at least you're aware that you need vitamins and minerals in your diet. What puzzles me is why popular interest in health and diet stops here, and doesn't go on to explain that *as important as what you put into your system are certain chemical balances achieved within the system.* These balances can mean the difference between health and illness; they can mean the difference between that aggravating bloated feeling and buckling up your belt a notch skinnier! Want to know more? Of course you do. Here's how to manipulate food chemistry to your advantage.

The Salt/Potassium Seesaw

Salt from a shaker, salt from the sea, the saltiness of tears—they all contain the familiar ion sodium. Potassium is another ion which, like sodium, carries a charge and moves in and out of cells via a sort of magnetic attraction.

So what, you say. Here's what: This snippet of a chemistry lesson bears directly on your well-being and your waistline. Sodium and potassium are the co-conspirators in water retention, for example. Take in more sodium than potassium, and you can retain excess water. Sodium drives body fluids into cells, plumping them up—and plumping *you* up.

The other end of the seesaw: Potassium helps keep water *out* of cells; it deflates what sodium inflates. You want as much potassium as sodium in your diet, is my point.

Together, sodium and potassium also choreograph such vital metabolic "dances" as muscle contractions and nerve cell transmissions. Too little or too much potassium, for instance, can result in heart rhythm disturbances. Too much sodium, meanwhile, can raise blood pressure in susceptible individuals. Here again, balance is vital.

Now, diet is a factor in the ebb and flow of sodium and potassium. You can perfect a do-it-yourself balancing act, if you know what you're doing. You do that by getting the same amount of potassium as you do sodium. Simple! Your diet can contain about four to five grams of each per day, without worrying about bloating. At these levels, sodium won't bloat you, and blood pressure should not be affected. Brilliant! The Palm Beach Diet achieves this ideal balance.

You might guess that the typical American diet is

lacking when it comes to this important balance of nutrients. The average American meal contains at least ten times as much sodium as potassium; this threatens blood pressure levels in those people who are salt-sensitive and also encourages water retention.

The Palm Beach Diet, then, bumps up potassium, and puts a lid on sodium. On the diet, your potassium comes from delectables such as avocado, almonds, spinach, raisins, and that star source of potassium—citrus fruit. Florida's native pride!

Warning: These health aids may be hazardous

You can also shape up your system's sodium/potassium status by avoiding a few so-called "health aids" that are quite popular now. That's right, *avoid* them. Such paraphernalia as home water softeners and salt substitutes actually can disrupt the body's ion balancing act.

Water-softening devices are installed into plumbing systems to encourage more lather from soaps. They act by removing calcium from hard water, making it less gritty. This *sounds* healthy, but removing minerals from drinking water may be health-*dumb*. Population studies show that people who live in hard-water areas have a lower incidence of death from coronary heart disease than do people who live in soft-water areas.

Not only is hard water desirable, then, but most water softeners introduce salt to the water to boot. Salt is used in exchange for calcium in most of these devices. Everyone over fifty should check that a home water softener does *not* use salt as a filtering agent.

The salt substitute is another good idea that can go wrong. These alternatives to table salt contain potassium. I agree that it's smart to reduce salt use as you grow older, to reduce potential risk of high blood pressure. And the use of potassium-based salt substitutes in moderation is perfectly fine. My concern is that these substitute products sometimes are seen as license to let loose a "snow" of seasoning all over the dinner plate. They're not: While most people just pass the excess potassium out in their urine, they can be dangerous if your kidneys are not up to par and if used with a heavy hand. This could create heart rhythm disturbances. (The taste alone should prohibit gourmands from overdoing. Let's just say it doesn't earn five stars.) Use salt substitutes in moderation.

While we're at the kitchen shelf, let's flash on another health product: vitamin C supplements. Even vitamin C tablets can be salty! If you take vitamin C supplements in the form of *sodium ascorbate,* you're getting sodium, or salt, along with the vitamin. If you insist on vitamin C supplements, choose one of vitamin C's many other forms.

> **Palm Beach Postscript:** People with kidney disease and anyone taking diuretics or potassium supplements must check with their doctor before starting on a low-salt, potassium-matching diet.

Keeping Phosphorus's Mitts Off Calcium

Let me keep you in suspense a moment before introducing you to phosphorus and calcium. In fact, let me take you to lunch instead—at the local fast-food chain.

When you order that fast-food cliché—a hamburger, French fries and a cola—just what are you getting? What did nature and modern processing put into the meal you're about to take out?

Good protein, yes, and iron to some degree. But you also are getting plenty of fat and the most health-threatening kind of fat—saturated animal fat. (You'll discover its liabilities a few pages ahead.) You also are ingesting cholesterol galore, calories through the roof, and at least seven teaspoons of sugar in most sweetened soft drinks. None of this is good for you. Remember this next time you reach for something you know isn't doing you any nutritional favors: Its appeal lasts a few taste-bud pleasing seconds; then it's over, all gone. Its consequences register much, much longer on your scales and in the body. In fact, let's track the digestive life of a fast-food lunch.

What's a Nosh Like You Doing in a Place Like This

Let's take a look specifically at fat. After all, fat is what you want to get rid of. Maybe a whiz-bang tour of "where fat winds up" will make you hesitate before reaching for your next helping of French fries!

To absorb fats, the body produces something called *bile salts.* The more meat, grease, milk, cream, etc., consumed per meal, the more bile salts produced in the liver. Certain bile salts have been implicated in cancer of the intestine. Already you see that fat is no friend of yours. (Even forgetting momentarily that it loans your middle the aura of an inner tube!)

Next, components of saturated fats get taken up by the liver, and packaged with proteins before shooting off into the bloodstream for various destinations. These fatty substances may go toward the construction of cell membranes; they may be claimed and used by the brain, which is almost all fatty substances. Then again, if you overdid on French fries, and ate fifty instead of five or so, you've got more fat in the bloodstream than you have productive uses for! This excess fat will be stored in your body. Everywhere. It only *seems* to all go to your stomach or hips. Eventually it might be used as energy—if you exercise more than you eat—but chances are it will remain "lying around" organs and under skin, burdening the system and ballooning your profile.

What else does our suddenly unappetizing lunch do? It delivers you more sodium than potassium. You want as much potassium as sodium, remember? This typical American meal also botches another important balance. This one involves phosphorus and calcium.

Phosphorus, like calcium, is a mineral found mainly in muscle and bone. The body needs some phosphorus in order to manufacture cell membranes, produce energy and activate vitamins, but it doesn't need Herculean amounts of phosphorus, which is where our all-American meal once again rates a thumbs-down. Hamburger meat and soda contain walloping amounts of phosphorus; they contain little calcium. This is significant because calcium is vital to people over fifty, and phosphorus inhibits calcium absorption.

A diet too high in meat can whammy your calcium status a second way, too: The high protein content of meat can encourage calcium *loss* from the body.

Age is a third strike against calcium status: According to a number of surveys, the mineral most often low in the diet of older Americans is calcium. In fact, most mature individuals are in what's called a "negative calcium balance," meaning they lose more calcium from bone than they absorb from their diet. The gradual loss of calcium is one reason we lose bone density as we grow older. This invites fractures, and loss of teeth later in life. It also can result in the disease known as *osteoporosis,* in which bone wastes to such a degree as to cause pain, disfigurement and disability.

Obviously, if adequate calcium can help prevent bone loss, your diet should be calcium-rich. Just as obvious: You should avoid excess phosphorus, because it compromises calcium status. And yet, the typical American diet contains three times as much phosphorus as calcium! Meat contains 20 to 30 times more phosphorus than calcium. Soft drinks are another challenge to healthy calcium/phosphorus balance: Many sodas contain five–ten times more—you guessed it—phosphorus than calcium. *Now you can begin to see how the eating pattern typical of the American adult invites nutritional imbalances, and threatens health.*

The ideal balance here is one milligram of calcium to every one milligram of phosphorus you consume. This ideal balance is difficult to achieve, though: As I mentioned earlier, many foods contain only small amounts of calcium, while phosphorus sometimes can seem omnipresent. On the Palm Beach Diet, the ratio between phosphorus and calcium is roughly 2½:1—not perfect, but still terrific. The more closely calcium levels approach phosphorus levels, the better.

You want your share of calcium for other reasons, too. A recent and intriguing observation: A calcium-high diet appears to have a quasi-protective effect against high blood pressure. No one is saying that a glass or two of milk a day will reverse high blood pressure, mind you. Or that not getting enough calcium will increase blood pressure. The case for calcium's effect on blood pressure is still being built. One speculation is that calcium somehow may defuse sodium's effect on blood pressure.

Calcium may also act as a slight hedge against heart disease. Although not conclusive, one study found that calcium supplements decreased cholesterol levels in elderly men and women.

Now you can see why your calcium/phosphorus balance is crucial—and why calcium is key.

Ideally, you should receive all your calcium from food. Practically, though, this is *tough.* Unless you're crazy about milk, cheese, yogurt, and other dairy products, you get less calcium than is optimal, now that you're fifty or more. To the rescue then comes the Palm Beach Diet's daily calcium supplements.

Now that you're on head-nodding terms with potassium, phosphorus and assorted microgoodies, let's return to what dieting is all about. Fat. Frumpy, infuriating fat.

Dangerous Fat vs. Safe Fat

The kind and amount of fat you eat throughout life can influence your health in later life. Your fat intake "profile," in fact, may even predict your vulnerability to certain health problems.

The Palm Beach Diet sees that your fat intake doesn't commit the typical American diet-crime of imbalance: either too much fat from meat and butter (most of us are guilty here) or too much fat from vegetable sources, mainly vegetable oils.

Fat is not all the same silhouette-shattering stuff. There are *saturated fats,* found mainly in meats, eggs and dairy products. (Saturated fats tend to harden at room temperature, should you need an identifying clue.) Then there are *polyunsaturated fats*—liquidy fats from vegetable sources. *Monounsaturated fats*—from fish, nuts, and olive oil, mainly—will be introduced later. The only difference between these substances, by the way, is the number of hydrogen atoms surrounding a cluster of carbon atoms! But what a difference a few hydrogen atoms can make to your health. . . .

The medical community has heaped criticism all over the fat-saturated American diet and has warned: Get too much saturated fat and you may wind up with heart disease or gallbladder disease.

Recognizing saturated fat as the insidious menace it is, many doctors have suggested limiting butter, eggs, cheeses, whole milk and cream in the diet. They recommend that you use polyunsaturated vegetable oils and vegetable-oil based margarines, in place of butter. These recommendations probably sound familiar to you: They have become standard medical advice. Recently, though, we've come to question whether polyunsaturated fats, such as those in vegetable oils, aren't without their health risks, too, when used in substantial amounts.

A diet high in polyunsaturated fats (the vegetable oil sort), appears to increase the risk of cancer, according to recent studies. While the final word isn't in yet, a diet very high in vegetable fat is probably risky.

What's going on? Researchers speculate that too much unsaturated vegetable fat interferes with the immune system, perhaps in two ways. *First:* Vegetable fats can soften cell membranes; this may make it easier for cancer-causing substances to invade cells. Second: Polyunsaturated fats also appear to make white blood cells less sticky. These white blood cells—the bloodstream's police force—then may literally lose their grip on bad-guy invaders! If the theory is true, it's easy to see how a case of "butter-fingers" could depress white blood cells' immune functioning.

What does all this mean to your diet? Find variety. You want a 1:1 ratio of saturated fat to unsaturated fat. You can have butter, in limited amounts, on the Palm Beach Diet; on the other hand, certain of the diet's quick recipes will call for vegetable oils. You'll be divvying up your fat "types," in other words. You also will be getting monounsaturated, or "safe," fat.

When it's your choice—butter, margarine or vegetable oil—how should you choose? Here's some help in a checklist of fats you can and cannot use on the Palm Beach Diet. (See chart on opposite page)

As I mentioned earlier, there's a third type of fat, *monounsaturated* fat. This particular "atom-family" of fat keeps pretty quiet. It doesn't increase risk of heart attack. It's not associated with cancer. In fact, to the best

Yes, in Moderation	Only Occasionally	Never
soft margarines	butter	hydrogenated margarines
corn oil		coconut oil
olive oil		palm oil
safflower oil		
sesame oil		
soybean oil		
peanut oil		

of our knowledge today, *monounsaturated* fat is the safest form of fat. It is not as likely as other fats to cause or aggravate health problems. It, therefore, is the fat *"of choice"* on the Palm Beach Diet. Good sources of monounsaturated fat are fish and nuts; you'll find plenty of both on the Palm Beach Diet.

Want more good news about fish? There are some populations which consume large quantities of fish; they seem to have a lower rate of coronary heart disease than the American population. A particular acid in fish may be one heart-protective hero here: *eicosapentaenoic acid* is its tongue-twisting name. Fish also is relatively low in cholesterol and in saturated fat, and high in monounsaturated fat. As I said, a low-cholesterol, low-saturated fat diet is desirable. For all these reasons, the Palm Beach Diet loves fish.

CHAPTER 6

Losing (Weight) Gracefully

So much for the workings and the maintenance of your "inner machinery." I may be wrong, but I suspect that the main reason you want to lose weight is to look better. It's important to know how a diet affects your health—but it isn't exactly *thrilling* to wade through a discussion on zinc or to knit your eyebrows over the functions of phosphorus! But you learned a lot, didn't you? Now, let's make you smile a lot.

Some diets involve a bit of "Catch-22": You diet to look better; yet, when you finish losing weight, you may look worse than when you began. We've all seen this happen to friends and acquaintances who diet. A week or so into their regimen, they begin to look as if the stock market crashed and their life savings were tied up in over-the-counter options. They look pale and sunken; they feel irritable and headache-y. They don't look great; they look gaunt. At this point, the weight loss hardly seems worth the torment.

Mature dieters can reap even grimmer rewards. Too often, the hallmark of a successful fifty-plus dieter is wrinkles and sags. It's sad but true. Fat is lost, but the skin—less elastic than it once was—doesn't shrink back fully.

Another dubious reward of dieting is lopsided nutritional status. When you're on diets more than you're off them, you may not be getting the vitamins and minerals you need. Once more, constant dieting places tremendous stress on the body. The result is that chronic dieting can accelerate the aging process.

No wonder so many people—especially older people—are discouraged about dieting. On many weight-loss plans, you just can't lose gracefully!

The Palm Beach Diet stacks the odds in your favor. Your looks won't suffer; you won't feel listless and lackluster. Why not? The Palm Beach Diet recognizes an important fact: *At your age, taking weight off too quickly can undermine your looks.* It's important that you aim for a weight loss of about two pounds a week on this or *any* diet.

A moderate diet pace at least partially ensures you against the wrinkling and sagging that can accompany rapid weight loss. When fat disappears steadily and slowly, the skin can better accommodate the change. This is really important if you're fifty or more.

At a moderate diet pace, you will not experience the biochemical trauma of rapid weight loss. In fact, on the Palm Beach Diet, skin tone may well improve, thanks to the wealth of nutrients, liquids and fiber that encourage elimination of toxins, and to exercise (which I'll discuss later).

This is the aspect of the diet which has won devotees: *While you lose weight, you gain vitality.*

My patients who shape up on the diet also discover something else. They are content to lose one to two pounds a week. They assume a certain smugness when they see others frantically trying to lose ten pounds in ten days. *They know that too fast too soon doesn't last.* I know I find many of the popular crash diets not only unhealthy, but almost embarrassing. What is an "adult" doing attempting to live only on pineapple, pecking at each chunk with grim determination? Why choose to survive on meat and ice cream—shades of the low-carbohydrate diets. You deserve better. You deserve real meals. And of course you want to look great without jeopardizing your health, as some diet plans can. Need convincing? Here we go, then, with a run-through of the popular diets, and why you shouldn't, at fifty or more, attempt them.

The Low-Carb Hoodwink

Many of the popular weight-loss plans are low-carbohydrate diets. They include the Atkins diet, the Complete Scarsdale Diet, the Stillman Quick Weight Loss Diet and the Calories Don't Count Diet. The Drinking Man's Diet is a soused version of the same.

What's at work here? In many cases, much of the weight loss dropped on these diet plans is water and muscle. Let's look at muscle loss first. Why does muscle get lost? Simple. Because there is not enough carbohydrate in the diet to provide energy, the body starts to break down its own tissue for energy. And loss of muscle helps defeat your dieting purpose in the long run. When you lose muscle, you limit your ability to burn fat.

Next: water loss. On a low-carbohydrate diet, you lose water and may become dehydrated.

The biological state of "ketosis"is touted as magical on the low-carbohydrate diets. Actually it is an unhealthy condition in which the body burns fat as fuel because its fuel of choice—sugars converted from food and stored as glycogen—is nowhere to be had. Alas, the body burns fat *incompletely*, however. You don't lose much fat during ketosis: At most you would lose one pound every one to two months. But ketosis does produce substances called ketones which wreak havoc with health; they can accumulate in the blood and interfere with important body functions, such as kidney function. Ketosis can also make dieters weak, irritable, headachey, dizzy and nauseous.

What else? Low-carbohydrate foods (such as meat and dairy products) tend to be high in fat. You learned in the last few chapters that the mature system shouldn't have to tolerate an excess of fat. A low-carbohydrate diet also can raise uric acid levels in the body. High uric acid levels are associated with gout.

Sorry to be such a spoil sport, but low-carbohydrate diets also tend to lack essential vitamins. The high-protein aspect of these diets may not benefit the mature system, either. Protein is wonderful—to a certain point. Protein overload, however, can burden the liver and the kidneys. It can cause dehydration. Gorging on unlimited amounts of meat also increases the excretion rate of calcium: Calcium should be a keystone, not a fatality, of a diet for older individuals.

Had enough? Good. Anyone fifty or over should look upon these diets as they look upon a tax audit—that is, as something to be avoided at all cost!

Beware Liquid Protein Plans

To my mind, liquid protein diets and formula diets are another case of grasping at straws.

Liquid protein diets generally are formulas, sometimes containing vitamins in addition to protein, which are substitutes for one, two or three meals a day. Even under a doctor's supervision, many are dangerous, especially if calories total no more than 500 a day. Some liquid protein diets have been associated with health crises and even death, and consequently have been taken off the market. Limited calorie liquid protein diets can result in ketosis, loss of potassium and heart rhythm disturbances.

The Cambridge Diet is one type of liquid protein diet. The federal Food and Drug Administration is investigating several cases associated with this diet in which acute illness required hospitalization.

Formula diets do make dieting simple but also boring. And since they are possibly dangerous, too, I suggest that you forget them as a weight-loss strategy!

Debunking the "Miracle" Food Myth

Perhaps it's papaya today and lima beans tomorrow. You probably know what I'm referring to: the sort of Johnny-one-note diet which claims that one food or one type of food has some sort of magical property. This "magic" food generally does one of two things, according to diet lore: Either it somehow prevents you from gaining weight while you eat up a storm or it "melts" fat off your body. My reaction: Fat chance!

Stop and think for just one second: How can a diet that limits you to one type of food provide all the micro-goodies you need? How can it maintain healthy biochemical balances? Even more puzzling is how any *food* can promise to take weight *off*.

The Beverly Hills Diet, for example, claims that fully digested food in essence can't get "stuck" in the body and become fat. Actually, the opposite is true. Digested food is absorbed; undigested food is eliminated and can't possibly make you fat.

Another premise of this diet involves fruit: Fruit is purported to contain enzymes which help digest other fattening foods. Sorry. Enzymes in any food you eat are destroyed immediately by stomach acids. Your body produces all the enzymes you need. What *is* true is that the diet can cause diarrhea, potassium deficiency and heart rhythm irregularities.

Ditch Your Diet Pills

Wouldn't it be nice and easy to take a pill that kept you slim and sleek, without endangering your health? Unfortunately, no such pill exists.

Many of the diet pills you can buy without a prescription contain something called *phenylpropanolamine*—mercifully referred to as PPA—as the active ingredient. Drugs containing PPA can cause serious complications, including high blood pressure, kidney failure, convulsions and psychotic reactions in otherwise healthy people. These diet pills are even more risky for people who already have high blood pressure, diabetes or heart, kidney or thyroid disease. A number of people over fifty may have one of these conditions and be unaware of it. All this is scary enough, but there's more.

Drugs containing PPA can interact dangerously with other drugs commonly taken by people over fifty. People who take a drug prescribed for arthritis and cramps, called Indocin, should make a special point not to use diet pills, for example. PPA can also be hazardous to women on hormones, because the two substances may work synergistically to raise blood pressure. My point is to avoid diet pills containing PPA if you're fifty or more—and I advise anyone under fifty to avoid them as well.

Forget About Fasting, Please

I once studied fasting at the Metabolic Unit of the University of Florida Medical School. I would never recommend fasting as a weight-loss method. Fasting is nothing short of starvation. It causes protein wasting from the heart, liver, kidneys, skin and muscles—from vital organs, in other words! Fasting diets also can cause weakness, dizziness, headaches, ketosis and attacks of gout. Even ulcerative colitis has resulted. In short, fasting is an extreme and dangerous way to lose weight.

You have your choice, then. You can take weight off rapidly, risking illness, or you can take it off at a reasonable but not frantic clip, and safeguard your health and your looks at the same time. It's your choice. *My* choice starts when you turn the page.

PART TWO

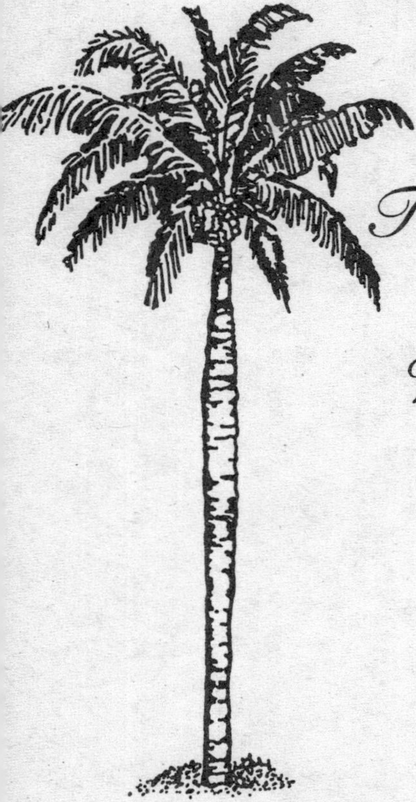

The 21 Days That Will Change Your Life

CHAPTER 7

The Palm Beach Diet

To start losing weight and to protect your health, follow the tempting meal plan here. It's that simple!

Follow it to the letter. Do not make substitutions other than those specified, or you may upset important nutritional balances. At the end of the week, you'll have lost up to two pounds of *fat.*

Of course, you may want to lose more than two pounds, total; perhaps a lot more. You can do so on the Palm Beach Diet—steadily, and at a moderate rate that won't jeopardize your health or your looks, now that you're fifty or more. You do that simply by staying on the diet until you reach your weight goal. Within a few weeks or a few months, you can drop pounds of fat that may have taken decades to accumulate!

Most people will want to start off on the "core" week of the diet, presented in this chapter. You can repeat the core week as often as you choose, or you can switch to "Easy Week"—seven days of super-simple and cost-conscious menus designed to make dieting especially convenient. You'll find "Easy Week" spelled out in Chapter 8. Or you may prefer to move on to "The Breakers" Week, Chapter 9.

Others of you may prefer to streamline your diet, and

stay with "Easy Week" start to finish. Note that you may repeat any week as often as desired. Once you have started one of the week-long plans, however, you are committed to that week: You cannot follow "Easy Week" on Monday and then switch to "The Breakers" Week on Tuesday, for example. Stay with a week until it is completed.

As you lose weight, you will be following meal plans which deliver still *more* nutritional bonuses. The Palm Beach Diet consists of, on average, 20–25 percent protein, approximately 30 percent fat, and 45–50 percent (mostly complex) carbohydrates! I consider this composition breakdown a healthy improvement on the mix of the typical American diet—roughly 20–25 percent protein, 35–40 percent fat, and 35–45 percent (mostly simple sugar) carbohydrates.

In addition, you'll be receiving on average 4–5 g. of sodium per day, maximum, and on average 200–300 mg. of cholesterol per day. These generally are considered safe and prudent levels. Many diet days, too, are substantially lower in both sodium and cholesterol. *Fiber,* meanwhile, is generously represented on the Palm Beach Diet: Most of it is found in foods which are complex carbohydrates—foods such as whole grain breads, cereals, vegetables and fruits. I'll praise the health and diet benefits of complex carbohydrates in later chapters. Know for now that you receive at the *very* least about 10 g. of fiber every day. That's good for you, and helpful toward your diet goal: Complex carbohydrates and fiber are more filling/less fattening, ounce for ounce, than many other foods.

The calorie count of each of the three weeks of the Palm Beach Diet is approximately 1000–1200 calories per day. As detailed in Chapter 6, this calorie level will ensure weight loss in most individuals, without inviting potential health problems associated with too-rapid weight loss.

The Palm Beach Diet is sugar-conscious, too. Sugar may appeal to a sweet tooth (until that sweet tooth decays, of course) but it is the ultimate high-calorie, low-nutrient food. In fact, sugar contains *no* nutrients whatsoever and it *can* raise blood insulin levels, which in turn can lower blood sugar levels and cause rebound hunger. Still, most Americans—accustomed to plenty of sugary foods in their diet—feel absolutely deprived if they can't have an occasional sweet treat. For this reason, you are allowed an occasional sweet dessert—lowfat ice cream, or sherbet, for instance—while dieting.

Ready, then? Here are the ground rules for the diet. Don't panic. They *look* far more complicated than they are! In a matter of days, they should become second nature.

The Palm Beach Diet Ground Rules

1. Take a multivitamin/mineral supplement every day.

Choose a multivitamin/mineral supplement which contains roughly the Recommended Daily Allowance (the amounts given below) for the following nutrients.

Vitamin A	5000 I.U.
Vitamin B_1 (Thiamine)	1–2 mg.
Vitamin B_6 (Pyridoxine)	2 mg.
Vitamin B_{12}	3 mcg.
Folic acid	400 mcg.
Vitamin C	60 mg.
Vitamin D	200 I.U.
Vitamin E	15 I.U.
Iron	10 mg.
Zinc	15 mg.
Calcium	0–200 mg.

The RDAs are printed on vitamin bottle labels and/or packing boxes.

Vitamin/mineral supplements meeting these requirements are widely available. Don't worry if your brand contains slightly more or less of these nutrients—as long as it contains each nutrient cited in amounts which approximate those above. It is also perfectly fine (and usual) for multivitamin/mineral supplements to contain other nutrients along with those listed above.

2. *Take a calcium supplement every day.*

The only nutrient listed above which is below the current Recommended Daily Allowance is calcium. And research suggests that you want *more* than the RDA of calcium if you're fifty or older. Therefore, you should take a calcium supplement every day.

The most inexpensive, and convenient, way to get extra calcium is calcium carbonate antacid tablets—but only those antacid tablets which are sodium-free, and which do *not* contain aluminum hydroxide (which encourages loss of phosphate, and calcium, from bone). Confusing? Not really. Two brands of antacids currently meet these requirements: Tums and Titralac. If you take five Tums or six Titralac a day, you are getting the same amount of calcium as is contained in a quart of milk—at a lower calorie and dollar cost. The ground rule, then: Take either five Tums or six Titralac a day.

If you take antacids, check with your doctor if you have kidney disease, kidney stones, a history of hypercalcemia (high blood calcium), drink a lot of milk, take vitamin D supplements or take calcium-blocking drugs. Also check with your doctor if you use theophylline, a drug used for breathing disorders. Antacids can increase the potency of the drug. Neither should antacids be taken together with the drug cimetidine (Tagamet is the brand name) prescribed for ulcers and other stomach conditions. Antacids can inactivate this drug.

Do not take more antacid tablets or calcium supplementation than is recommended here. Large doses of calcium carbonate antacid tablets can compromise iron, phosphorus and vitamin B_1, and can turn the blood dangerously alkaline. "Megadosing" on antacids also can cause fluid retention. Don't overdo.

3. Drink six glasses of water a day.

Choose from tap water, mineral water, seltzer water and sparkling water. While diet soda is not recommended on the diet, you may, if you choose to, substitute one 12-ounce can of diet soda for a glass of water per day.

4. Do not use table salt for cooking or for flavoring. Use salt substitutes in moderation only.

5. Do not use sugar.

While you'll have an occasional sweet "treat" while dieting, do not *add* sugar to foods. You may use the sugar substitutes Equal, NutraSweet and sorbitol in moderation. I prefer you avoid saccharin, if possible.

6. Choose whole grain breads.

The label will indicate as much. Look for the notations "whole grain" or "whole wheat." Breads containing preservatives are okay.

7. Use fresh fruits, vegetables and fish when possible.

If fresh foods are unavailable, frozen is second best. Canned foods should be your last choice. All canned food should be as sugar- and sodium-low as possible; rinse in cold water prior to using.

8. You may use soft margarines, corn oil, olive oil, safflower oil, sesame oil, soybean oil and peanut oil.

You may not use hydrogenated (generally hard) margarines, coconut oil or palm oil. Butter should be used only when specified on the diet.

9. Choose raw and unsalted nuts.

10. Measure foods uncooked.

When the diet calls for ½ cup spinach, for instance, or 2 ounces of pasta, or 5 ounces of fish, that's the measure of weight of the food *before* cooking.

The Palm Beach Diet: Core Week Menus and Recipes

MONDAY

Calories: 1100–1200

BREAKFAST

Oatmeal (⅓ cup before cooking) topped with
1 tablespoon almonds
and 1 tablespoon chopped dates
(you may substitute raisins for dates)
¼ cup skim milk
Coffee or tea, with skim milk
and/or sugar substitute, if desired

MID-MORNING SNACK

1 piece of fresh fruit—your choice
Multivitamin/mineral supplement

LUNCH

*Palm Beach Salad** (* indicates that recipe follows)
in a medium whole-wheat pita pocket
1 ounce Cheddar cheese
Coffee or tea, with skim milk
and/or sugar substitute, if desired

DINNER

*Grouper Baked with Artichoke Hearts**
(you may substitute any white fish for grouper)
*Spinach Fettuccine with Garlic**
1 cup steamed broccoli
2 pear halves, sliced in ¼ cup orange juice,
and seasoned with ground ginger
Coffee or tea, with skim milk
and/or sugar substitute, if desired

Remember your 6 glasses of water and your calcium supplement.

MONDAY RECIPES

PALM BEACH SALAD

Equal parts alfalfa sprouts (or bean sprouts) and watercress
½ cup mushrooms
½ cup asparagus

Toss ingredients together with 2 tablespoons of either Palm Beach Dressing #1 or Palm Beach Dressing #2.

PALM BEACH DRESSING #1

1 small clove garlic, crushed
1 tablespoon mustard powder
¼ cup boiling water
¼ teaspoon dried dill (or 1 tablespoon fresh dill)
⅓ cup red wine vinegar
½ cup tightly packed fresh parsley
1 cup plain yogurt

Combine first 6 ingredients in a blender or food processor; process until smooth. (By-hand method: Finely chop the parsley and combine with first 5 ingredients.) Transfer to a container; stir in the yogurt.

Makes about 1½ cups dressing, about 6 calories per tablespoon. Dressing keeps in the refrigerator up to 2 weeks.

PALM BEACH DRESSING #2

1 teaspoon vegetable oil
1 clove garlic, cut into quarters
½ teaspoon dried basil
¼ teaspoon dried oregano
⅛ teaspoon dried thyme
⅛ teaspoon black pepper
Pinch cayenne pepper (optional)
1 cup tomato juice
1 tablespoon cornstarch
¼ cup red wine vinegar

In a small saucepan, combine oil, garlic, herbs and pepper. Cook over medium heat for 2 minutes, then stir in tomato juice. Mix cornstarch and vinegar in a measuring cup; stir until smooth. Stir cornstarch mixture into saucepan. Heat to boiling; boil 1 minute. Cool to room temperature, then store covered in refrigerator, up to 2 weeks. Makes about 1¼ cups, about 7 calories per tablespoon.

GROUPER BAKED WITH ARTICHOKE HEARTS

- 1 teaspoon margarine
- 3 ounces filet of grouper (or other white fish)
- ½ cup chopped tomato
- 1 tablespoon parsley
- ¼ teaspoon dried basil (or 1 tablespoon fresh basil)
- 4 artichoke hearts
- ½ cup sliced mushrooms
- 1 small clove garlic, crushed

Heat oven to 400° F. Use half of the margarine to grease a small ovenproof casserole or gratin dish. Place fish in casserole; top with remaining margarine, and remaining ingredients. Cover the casserole with aluminum foil as tightly as possible. Bake for about 8 minutes, until done.

SPINACH FETTUCCINE WITH GARLIC

- 3 ounces spinach fettuccine
- 1 teaspoon margarine
- 1 small clove garlic, crushed
- 1 tablespoon chopped or slivered almonds
- Several grindings black pepper

Bring 2 quarts of water to boiling in a small saucepan. Add fettuccine; cook to desired doneness. *Before draining fettuccine, remove ¼ cup of the cooking water from the pan; set aside.* Add margarine and garlic to the saucepan with the reserved cooking water. Toss over medium heat for 1–2 minutes so that the fettuccine absorbs some of the water. Add almonds and ground pepper to taste.

TUESDAY

Calories: 1000–1100

BREAKFAST

One 4-inch buckwheat pancake
(commercially prepared batter is fine)
½ cup fresh fruit
Coffee or tea, with skim milk
and/or sugar substitute, if desired

MID-MORNING SNACK

Small (1½ ounces) box of raisins
Multivitamin/mineral supplement

LUNCH

Crabmeat and citrus sandwich:
A medium whole-wheat pita pocket stuffed with
½ cup crabmeat, 2 teaspoons diet mayonnaise,
segments of half an orange, coarsely chopped
Coffee or tea, with skim milk
and/or sugar substitute, if desired

DINNER

*Quick Chicken Sauté**
½ cup brown rice tossed with ½ ounce cashews and parsley
½ cup lima beans
1 piece of fresh fruit—your choice
Coffee or tea, with skim milk
and/or sugar substitute, if desired

Remember your 6 glasses of water and your calcium supplement.

TUESDAY RECIPES

QUICK CHICKEN SAUTÉ

1 teaspoon vegetable oil
3 ounces boneless chicken breast, cut into thin strips
1 small clove garlic, crushed
½ cup red pepper, cut into thin strips
½ cup thinly sliced onion
½ cup sliced mushrooms
Pinch cayenne pepper (optional)

Heat the oil in a nonstick skillet over medium heat. Add the chicken strips; cook until browned on all sides, about 3 minutes. Remove chicken; set aside. Add remaining ingredients to skillet; cook over medium heat for 3–4 minutes, until onion is softened. Return chicken to skillet; heat through for another minute and serve.

WEDNESDAY

Calories: 1100–1200

BREAKFAST

½ cup grapefruit juice
1 poached egg on 1 slice whole grain bread or toast
1 teaspoon butter
4 asparagus spears
Coffee or tea, with skim milk
and/or sugar substitute, if desired

MID-MORNING SNACK

1 piece of fresh fruit—your choice
Multivitamin/mineral supplement

LUNCH

*Chicken Chutney Salad**
in a medium whole-wheat pita pocket
Coffee or tea, with skim milk
and/or sugar substitute, if desired

DINNER

*Spaghetti Primavera**
½ cup low-fat ice cream, or ice milk, sprinkled with
1 teaspoon coconut
Coffee or tea, with skim milk
and/or sugar substitute, if desired

Remember your 6 glasses of water and your calcium supplement.

WEDNESDAY RECIPES

CHICKEN CHUTNEY SALAD

Mix together 3 ounces of boneless cooked chicken, 2 teaspoons diet mayonnaise, 1 tablespoon mango chutney, 1 sliced apple and 1 tablespoon chopped almonds. Serve stuffed in a whole-wheat pita pocket.

SPAGHETTI PRIMAVERA

Cook 2 ounces of spaghetti according to package directions. Drain. Toss spaghetti with 2 cups cooked, mixed vegetables (fresh or frozen), and 1 teaspoon margarine, 1 teaspoon dried basil, 1 small clove garlic, crushed.

THURSDAY

Calories: 1000–1100

BREAKFAST

½ grapefruit
½ cup bran cereal topped with 2 ounces chopped dates
(you may substitute raisins for dates)
1 cup skim milk
Coffee or tea, with skim milk
and/or sugar substitute, if desired

MID-MORNING SNACK

1 piece of fresh fruit—your choice
Multivitamin/mineral supplement

LUNCH

*Paradise Salad**
Roll (you may substitute 1 slice whole grain bread for roll)
Coffee or tea, with skim milk
and/or sugar substitute, if desired

DINNER

*Shrimp Scampi** (you may substitute a commercially prepared frozen fish diet meal, up to 350 calories, for Shrimp Scampi, rice and broccoli)
½ cup long grain and wild rice
¾ cup steamed broccoli
4 ounces sherbet
Coffee or tea, with skim milk
and/or sugar substitute, if desired

Remember your 6 glasses of water and your calcium supplement.

THURSDAY RECIPES

PARADISE SALAD

Toss together raw spinach (as desired), 3 teaspoons cashews, ½ cup tangerine sections, 4 artichoke hearts, and raw onion rings to taste. Dress with 2 tablespoons either Palm Beach Dressing #1 or #2 (p. 76).

SHRIMP SCAMPI

1 teaspoon butter or margarine
1 small clove garlic, crushed
1 teaspoon rosemary
1 tablespoon lemon juice
Several grindings of black pepper
4 ounces shelled shrimp

Heat the butter or margarine in a nonstick skillet over medium heat. Add the next four ingredients to the skillet; distribute evenly over the surface of the skillet. Add the shrimp and cook for 5 minutes, until shrimp are cooked.

FRIDAY

Calories: 1000–1100

BREAKFAST

½ cup grapefruit juice
1 bran muffin
1 teaspoon butter or margarine
Coffee or tea, with skim milk
and/or sugar substitute, if desired

MID-MORNING SNACK

Small (1½ ounces) box of raisins
Multivitamin/mineral supplement

LUNCH

½ cantaloupe filled with ½ cup low-fat cottage cheese, sprinkled with chopped chives, served with a twist of lime
Coffee or tea, with skim milk and/or sugar substitute, if desired

DINNER

*Veal Piccata**
½ cup brown rice
½ cup snow peas (you may substitute green for snow peas)
½ cup steamed carrots tossed with parsley
½ cup low-fat ice cream, or ice milk, sprinkled with 1 teaspoon coconut
Coffee or tea, with skim milk and/or sugar substitute, if desired

Remember your 6 glasses of water and your calcium supplement.

FRIDAY RECIPES

VEAL PICCATA

3 ounces veal (*you may substitute skinless chicken breast*), pounded to a ⅛-inch thickness
1 teaspoon flour
1 teaspoon butter or margarine
2 tablespoons dry white wine
2 teaspoons lemon juice
Several grindings of black pepper

Sprinkle meat with flour. Heat ½ teaspoon of the butter or margarine in a nonstick skillet over medium-high heat. Add meat; cook about 2 minutes each side. Remove meat from skillet; keep warm. Add wine and lemon juice to skillet; simmer 1 minute. Add remaining ½ teaspoon butter or margarine, and black pepper. Pour sauce over meat and serve.

SATURDAY

Calories: 1000–1100

BREAKFAST

1 ounce Nova Scotia salmon and ½ ounce cream cheese on a bagel (you may substitute chopped liver for salmon)
Coffee or tea, with skim milk and/or sugar substitute, if desired

MID-MORNING SNACK

¾ cup plain yogurt sprinkled with 1 teaspoon coconut
Multivitamin/mineral supplement

LUNCH

*Scallop Salad** (you may substitute a commercially prepared frozen fish diet meal, up to 300 calories, for Scallop Salad)
Coffee or tea, with skim milk and/or sugar substitute, if desired

DINNER

*Pompano en Papillote** (you may substitute any dark fish such as mackerel, snapper, bluefish for pompano)
1 baked potato
2 broiled tomato halves

Coffee or tea, with skim milk
and/or sugar substitute, if desired

Remember your 6 glasses of water and your calcium supplement.

SATURDAY RECIPES

SCALLOP SALAD

Gently poach 2 ounces of bay (small) scallops. Let cool. Toss scallops with 4 artichoke hearts, 3 tablespoons prepared croutons, and salad greens of your choice. Serve dressed with either 2 tablespoons Palm Beach Dressing #1 or #2 (p. 76).

POMPANO EN PAPILLOTE

Parchment paper (or heavy brown paper)
1 teaspoon butter or margarine
3 ounces pompano (or other dark fish)
1 tablespoon chopped fresh dill (or ¼ teaspoon dried dill)
1 tablespoon chopped scallions
1 tablespoon chopped parsley
Several grindings of black pepper
Lemon wedge

Heat oven to 400° F. Cut a dinner plate-size circle of parchment paper or heavy brown paper. (Do not use paper bags; some are chemically treated.) Fold in half. Unfold and smear one half with ½ teaspoon butter or margarine, leaving a 1-inch border all around. Place fish on greased side of the center fold.

In a small bowl combine the remaining ½ teaspoon butter or margarine, dill, scallions, parsley and pepper; mix well. Spread over fish. Fold free half of the paper over the fish, and staple closed. Place the package on a baking sheet and bake for 10 minutes. Remove fish package from oven, and with a sharp knife or scissors, cut an "X" in the top of the paper. Tear back paper and serve fish with lemon wedge.

SUNDAY

Calories: 1000–1100

BREAKFAST

½ grapefruit
1 bran muffin
1 teaspoon butter or margarine
Coffee or tea, with skim milk
and/or sugar substitute, if desired

BRUNCH

Egg Florentine: one poached egg on a bed of spinach
(½ cup after cooking), sprinkled with nutmeg
¾ cup strawberries
4 ounces dry champagne (you may substitute a Bloody Mary
or a "Virgin Mary" for champagne)
Coffee or tea, with skim milk
and/or sugar substitute, if desired

MID-DAY SNACK

12 raw almonds
Multivitamin/mineral supplement

DINNER

*Turkey and Vegetable Curry**
½ cup brown rice
1 tablespoon mango chutney
Coffee or tea, with skim milk
and/or sugar substitute, if desired

Remember your 6 glasses of water and your calcium supplement.

SUNDAY RECIPES

TURKEY AND VEGETABLE CURRY

SERVES 2

1 teaspoon vegetable oil
6 ounces boneless turkey meat (fresh or frozen turkey cutlet), cut into 1-inch chunks
1 cup chopped onion
1 cup sliced carrots (2 medium)
1 clove garlic, crushed
2 teaspoons curry powder
½ teaspoon ground cumin
Pinch of black pepper
1 cup sliced zucchini (1 small)
½ cup peas
½ cup chopped tomato
1 tablespoon chopped almonds
¾ cup water
½ teaspoon cornstarch
¼ cup skim milk

Heat the oil in a nonstick skillet; add the turkey and cook over medium-high heat, stirring occasionally until browned on all sides, about 3 minutes. Remove turkey from skillet; set aside. Add onion, carrots and garlic and cook, covered, for 5 minutes, until the onion is softened. Add the curry, cumin, and pepper; cook, stirring, for 1 minute. Add the remaining vegetables and the almonds, and the water; simmer, covered, for 5 more minutes. Combine the cornstarch and milk in a small bowl; stir until smooth. Stir into skillet, and heat mixture to boiling. Return turkey pieces to the skillet and heat through. Serve over brown rice.

This dish can be made the day before, if desired.

CHAPTER 8

The Palm Beach Diet—Easy Week

Here's the super-simple plan that nearly makes itself—a week of menus that is easy and economical. Easy Week is a favorite among people who wish to diet without frills. Like the Palm Beach Diet "core" week, it's optimally balanced for health. Enjoy!

MONDAY

Calories: 1000–1100

BREAKFAST

½ cup grapefruit juice
An 8-ounce tub of plain, coffee, lemon or vanilla low-fat yogurt
1 slice whole wheat toast
1 teaspoon margarine
Coffee or tea, with skim milk and/or sugar substitute, if desired

MID-MORNING SNACK

1 piece of fresh fruit—your choice
Multivitamin/mineral supplement

LUNCH

Cup of vegetable soup (low-sodium if possible)
Hard roll filled with 1 ounce Cheddar cheese, sliced tomato,
lettuce and 1 teaspoon diet mayonnaise
Coffee or tea, with skim milk
and/or sugar substitute, if desired

DINNER

3 ounces broiled white fish (such as grouper, cod, sole)
½ cup peas
1 cup steamed spinach
1 tomato, sliced
Whole wheat roll
1 teaspoon butter or margarine
Coffee or tea, with skim milk
and/or sugar substitute, if desired

Remember your 6 glasses of water and your calcium supplement.

TUESDAY

Calories: 1000–1100

BREAKFAST

½ cup grapefruit juice
Oatmeal (⅓ cup before cooking) topped with 2 teaspoons raisins
½ cup skim milk
Coffee or tea, with skim milk
and/or sugar substitute, if desired

MID-MORNING SNACK

1 piece of fresh fruit—your choice
Multivitamin/mineral supplement

LUNCH

*Health Salad to Go**
(you may substitute a garden salad of lettuce, tomato, cucumber, parsley and 1 ounce American cheese with low-calorie dressing, for Health Salad to Go)
Whole wheat roll
1 teaspoon margarine
Coffee or tea, with skim milk
and/or sugar substitute, if desired

DINNER

3 ounces broiled white fish (such as grouper, cod, sole)
*Palm Beach Slaw**
1 baked potato
½ cup green beans
Coffee or tea, with skim milk
and/or sugar substitute, if desired

Remember your 6 glasses of water and your calcium supplement.

TUESDAY RECIPES

HEALTH SALAD TO GO

This portable salad can be made at home and taken to work in a plastic-lidded container.

½ cup raw sliced zucchini
½ cup chick peas, drained
1 tomato, sliced
Chopped fresh parsley (or parsley flakes)

Combine all ingredients and toss with 2 tablespoons Palm Beach Dressing #1 (p. 76).

PALM BEACH SLAW

1 cup shredded cabbage
1 small carrot, shredded
1 tablespoon raisins
⅛ teaspoon caraway seeds
2 tablespoons plain yogurt (*you may substitute diet mayonnaise for yogurt*)

Combine all ingredients in a bowl; toss until coated with the yogurt.

WEDNESDAY

Calories: 1000–1100

BREAKFAST

¾ cup orange juice
1 bran muffin
1 teaspoon margarine
Coffee or tea, with skim milk
and/or sugar substitute, if desired

MID-MORNING SNACK

1 piece of fresh fruit—your choice
Multivitamin/mineral supplement

LUNCH

Tuna sandwich: 3 ounces water-packed tuna, 1 teaspoon diet mayonnaise, 1 tablespoon chopped onion on 2 slices whole wheat bread

Coffee or tea, with skim milk
and/or sugar substitute, if desired

MID-AFTERNOON SNACK

10 raw almonds

DINNER

*Steamed Vegetables**
½ cup brown rice
2 teaspoons mango chutney
*Ambrosia** (you may substitute 1 cup fruit cocktail canned in natural juices for Ambrosia)
Coffee or tea, with skim milk
and/or sugar substitute, if desired

Remember your 6 glasses of water and your calcium supplement.

WEDNESDAY RECIPES

STEAMED VEGETABLES

½ cup carrots, cut into ⅛-inch rounds
1 medium onion, sliced
1½ cups coarsely chopped broccoli
1 cup fresh bean sprouts

Heat 1 inch of water in a saucepan large enough to hold a vegetable steamer. Arrange vegetables in steamer: carrots on bottom, onion in the middle, broccoli on top. Place steamer into the pan when water begins to boil; cover and steam for about 5 minutes.

Add bean sprouts to the steamer just at the point the broccoli is cooked yet crisp. Steam vegetables 1 minute more, until bean sprouts are heated through. Transfer vegetables to a serving plate with brown rice and 2 teaspoons mango chutney.

AMBROSIA

1 orange, broken into segments
½ cup pineapple, packed in natural or light juices
1 tablespoon coconut

Combine all ingredients in a small bowl; toss well.

THURSDAY

Calories: 1000–1100

BREAKFAST

*Southern Smoothie**

MID-MORNING SNACK

1 corn muffin, plain
Coffee or tea, with skim milk
and/or sugar substitute, if desired
Multivitamin/mineral supplement

LUNCH

*Palm Beach Portable Salad**
Coffee or tea, with skim milk
and/or sugar substitute, if desired

MID-AFTERNOON SNACK

1 piece of fresh fruit—your choice

DINNER

Minute Steak with Mushrooms: 4-ounce cubed minute steak sautéed with ¾ cup mushrooms and ½ cup sliced onion in 2 teaspoons oil (you may substitute a commercially prepared frozen diet meal, up to 350 calories, for Minute Steak with Mushrooms, potato and zucchini)
1 small baked potato
1 cup steamed zucchini
Coffee or tea, with skim milk and/or sugar substitute, if desired

THURSDAY RECIPES

SOUTHERN SMOOTHIE

In a blender or food processor, combine ½ cup plain low-fat yogurt, 1 banana, ½ cup orange juice, 1 ice cube. Blend until smooth.

PALM BEACH PORTABLE SALAD

This portable salad can be made at home and taken to work in a plastic-lidded container:

- 1 cup raw spinach
- 1 tangerine, sectioned
- 2 ounces mild cheese
- Onion rings to taste

Combine all ingredients and toss with 2 tablespoons Palm Beach Dressing #1 (p. 76).

FRIDAY

Calories: 1000–1100

BREAKFAST

½ cup orange juice
1 slice raisin bread, toasted, sprinkled with cinnamon
1 teaspoon margarine or butter
Coffee or tea, with skim milk
and/or sugar substitute, if desired

MID-MORNING SNACK

1 piece of fresh fruit—your choice
Multivitamin/mineral supplement

LUNCH

3-ounce broiled hamburger patty,
on lettuce, with 1 slice tomato
½ cup green beans tossed with 6 almonds, slivered
Small luncheon roll
Coffee or tea, with skim milk
and/or sugar substitute, if desired

DINNER

3 ounces broiled or baked chicken
1 cup pasta spirals with 2 tablespoons Parmesan cheese
1 tomato, sliced
¼ cup sorbet or sherbet
Coffee or tea, with skim milk
and/or sugar substitute, if desired

Remember your 6 glasses of water and your calcium supplement.

SATURDAY

Calories: 1000–1100

BREAKFAST

½ cup grapefruit juice
½ cup bran cereal, sprinkled with 2 tablespoons raisins
½ cup skim milk
Coffee or tea, with skim milk
and/or sugar substitute, if desired

MID-MORNING

Multivitamin/mineral supplement

LUNCH

*Paradise Salad** (Recipe page 82—you may substitute a commercially prepared frozen diet meal, up to 300 calories, for Paradise Salad)
Coffee or tea, with skim milk
and/or sugar substitute, if desired

DINNER

4 ounces broiled fish—your choice
1 small sweet potato
½ cup steamed zucchini
1 cup sliced cucumber
Lime wedges
3-inch square of uniced angel-food cake
Coffee or tea, with skim milk
and/or sugar substitute, if desired

Remember your 6 glasses of water and your calcium supplement.

SUNDAY

Calories: 1000–1100

BREAKFAST

*Three-Fruit Favorite**
½ cup plain yogurt
Multivitamin/mineral supplement
Coffee or tea, with skim milk
and/or sugar substitute, if desired

SUNDAY DINNER

*Southern Ginger Pork**
1 small sweet potato
½ cup green beans
Coffee or tea, with skim milk
and/or sugar substitute, if desired

SUPPER

Turkey sandwich: 2 ounces turkey, lettuce, 1 teaspoon diet mayonnaise on 2 slices whole wheat bread
½ cup low-fat ice cream, or ice milk, sprinkled with 1 teaspoon coconut
Coffee or tea, with skim milk
and/or sugar substitute, if desired

Remember your 6 glasses of water and your calcium supplement.

SUNDAY RECIPES

THREE-FRUIT FAVORITE

¾ strawberries, fresh or frozen
1 banana, sliced
1 orange, sectioned

Combine all ingredients in a serving bowl.

SOUTHERN GINGER PORK

2 teaspoons oil
2 ounces lean boneless pork, cut into ¼-inch slices
1 teaspoon grated fresh ginger (or ¼ teaspoon ground ginger)
1 clove garlic, crushed
⅓ cup orange juice
½ teaspoon cornstarch
1 orange, peeled and cut into ¼-inch rounds

Heat the oil in a nonstick skillet over medium-high heat. Add the pork; cook 3 minutes. Turn the pork; cook 3 to 4 minutes more. Remove pork from skillet.

Add the ginger and garlic to skillet; cook 1 minute. Mix the orange juice with the cornstarch; pour into skillet. Add pork slices and orange slices to skillet; toss to coat.

CHAPTER 9

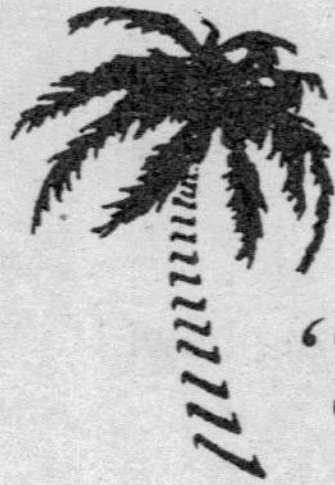

The Palm Beach Diet—"The Breakers" Week

"The Breakers," of course, is the legendary Palm Beach hotel—a bastion of elegance and perhaps the island's best-known landmark. Long famous for its spectacular and inventive menus, the Breakers remains today a prime location for society balls and stylish dining.

The hotel's Florentine dining room and elaborate kitchens are headed by executive chef Karl Ronaszeki, a native of Budapest, Hungary, and a winner of the Five Star Award from the Classical Gourmet Society. It's with pleasure and local pride that I present Chef Ronaszeki's contribution to the Palm Beach Diet—a week of stunning yet low-calorie menus which perfectly illustrate the appeal of today's "new cuisine."

MONDAY

Calories: 1000–1100

BREAKFAST

½ cup orange juice
1 slice grilled bacon
1 grilled tomato
1 slice whole wheat toast
1 teaspoon whipped sweet butter or margarine
Tea or coffee with sugar substitute, if desired

MID-MORNING SNACK

½ cup fresh raspberries (or any berry in season)
¾ cup skim milk

(Multivitamin/mineral supplement per the Palm Beach Diet)

LUNCH

½ pink grapefruit
6 medium shrimp, peeled and cooked, served on 2 slices of cucumber, 2 slices of tomato and leaves of Boston lettuce
Dressing: 1 teaspoon salad oil, 1 teaspoon red wine vinegar
2 slices of melba toast
¾ cup skim milk
Coffee or iced tea with sugar substitute, if desired

DINNER

¾ cup consomme (low-salt if possible) with
6 asparagus spears (poached or steamed)
broiled veal chop
1 medium boiled potato
1 medium grilled tomato
¼ cup broccoli
¼ cup white wine diluted with seltzer water
½ pear
10 grapes
Coffee or tea with sugar substitute, if desired

(6 glasses of water and calcium supplement per the Palm Beach Diet)

TUESDAY

Calories: 1000–1100

BREAKFAST

½ cup shredded wheat cereal with ¾ cup skim milk
½ medium apple
1 slice rye toast
½ teaspoon whipped sweet butter
Coffee or tea with sugar substitute, if desired

MID-MORNING SNACK

½ cantaloupe
Glass of seltzer water with twist of lemon
(Multivitamin/mineral supplement per the Palm Beach Diet)

LUNCH

*Broiled Filet of Sole Francaise**
½ cup steamed zucchini
Coffee or iced tea with sugar substitute, if desired

DINNER

½ cup lobster meat on lettuce leaves
Dressing: 1 teaspoon lemon juice, 1 teaspoon salad oil
2–3 ounces lean lamb chop, grilled
1 medium baked potato
½ cup cooked new peas
1 dietetic bread stick
½ cup lemon sorbet or sherbet
Coffee or tea with sugar substitute, if desired

(*6 glasses of water and calcium supplement per the Palm Beach Diet*)

TUESDAY RECIPES

BROILED FILET OF SOLE FRANCAISE

1 teaspoon margarine
2 ounces filet of sole
Pepper to taste
Juice of ¼ lemon

Egg wash:
1 egg
2 teaspoons milk diluted with 3 teaspoons water

Preheat a nonstick skillet. Heat margarine in the pan; dip filet of sole in egg wash and place sole in skillet. Sauté each side until golden brown, approximately 3 minutes per side. Pepper to taste. Add lemon juice; remove from flame. Serve with steamed zucchini.

WEDNESDAY

Calories: 1000–1100

BREAKFAST

¾ cup fresh orange juice
Egg-white omelet Florentine made with: two egg whites, ¼ cup chopped and cooked spinach, ½ teaspoon butter and garlic and pepper to taste
1 slice whole wheat toast
½ teaspoon whipped sweet butter
Coffee or tea with sugar substitute, if desired

MID-MORNING SNACK

10 raw almonds
Glass of seltzer water with twist of lime
(*Multivitamin/mineral supplement per the Palm Beach Diet*)

LUNCH

6 oysters on half-shell with juice of ½ lemon
Tropical fruit salad platter:
¼ cup diced watermelon
½ cup tangerine segments
¼ cup diced cantaloupe
¼ cup fresh pineapple—diced
¾ cup plain low-fat yogurt
3 melba toast rounds
Coffee or iced tea with sugar substitute, if desired

DINNER

1 cup clear consomme (*low-salt if possible*)
*Coquille Calloise**
3 dietetic bread sticks

¼ cup sorbet or sherbet
Coffee or tea with sugar substitute, if desired

(6 glasses of water and calcium supplement per the Palm Beach Diet)

WEDNESDAY RECIPES

COQUILLE CALLOISE

½ cup steamed leek
Pepper to taste
Juice of ½ lemon
1 teaspoon margarine
1 5-ounce lobster tail
3 Sea scallops
1 teaspoon white wine
½ cup mixed julienne vegetables (such as celery, carrot, zucchini, parsnip—well blanched and drained)

Place ½ cup steamed leek in blender and puree. Season with pepper to taste. Add half of the lemon juice. Place ¼ teaspoon margarine in puree; blend well. Set aside and keep hot.

Place remaining margarine in a sauté pan. Preheat. Remove tail meat from lobster shell. Score tail lengthwise. Add lobster tail to the pan. Sauté both sides of lobster tail, and then add scallops to the pan. Season contents lightly with pepper and remaining lemon juice. Add the wine and cook, covered, 3 minutes.

Place leek puree at the center of a plate and surround the puree with julienne vegetables. Top the leek puree with the lobster tail (red side up) and the scallops.

THURSDAY

Calories: 1000–1100

BREAKFAST

¾ cup fresh pineapple juice
1 prepared waffle with 3 teaspoons dietetic syrup
¼ cup blackberries or blueberries
Coffee or tea with sugar substitute, if desired

MID-MORNING SNACK

3 medium plums
Glass of mineral water with twist of lemon
(Multivitamin/mineral supplement per the Palm Beach Diet)

LUNCH

Cup of clear broth (low-sodium if possible)
*Poached Salmon Parisienne**
1 matzo
½ cup raspberry sorbet or sherbet
Coffee or tea with sugar substitute, if desired

DINNER

Salad of Bibb lettuce and 2 tomato slices
Dressing of 1 teaspoon lemon juice and 1 teaspoon salad oil
*Filet Mignon Gourmand**
Coffee or tea with sugar substitute, if desired

(6 glasses of water and calcium supplement per the Palm Beach Diet)

THURSDAY RECIPES

POACHED SALMON PARISIENNE

Serve a 3-ounce poached salmon filet with 2 cucumber slices, 2 tomato slices, 2 large and boiled asparagus spears, Bibb lettuce and 1 teaspoon diet mayonnaise. Garnish with lemon wedges and finely chopped dill.

FILET MIGNON GOURMAND

1 3-ounce filet
Pepper to taste
2 whole fresh mushrooms
1 teaspoon margarine
¼ cup cooked summer squash
¼ cup cooked zucchini
1 medium grilled tomato
1 teaspoon finely chopped shallots
¼ teaspoon finely chopped fresh parsley
2 teaspoons red wine

Season filet with pepper to taste; broil to medium doneness.

Lightly sauté mushrooms in ½ teaspoon margarine. In same pan, sauté summer squash, zucchini and grilled tomato. Season lightly with pepper. Remove from flame and keep hot.

Place filet on center of a plate; surround with vegetables. Place remaining ½ teaspoon margarine in sauté pan; add shallots. Sauté lightly; add pepper to taste. Add chopped parsley and the wine; cover and cook 2 minutes. Pour sauce over the filet.

FRIDAY

Calories: 1000–1100

BREAKFAST

⅔ cup apple juice
½ cup bran cereal with ¾ cup skim milk
Coffee or tea with sugar substitute, if desired

MID-MORNING SNACK

½ honeydew melon
Glass of seltzer water with twist of lemon
(Multivitamin/mineral supplement per the Palm Beach Diet)

LUNCH

½ grapefruit
*Breast of Chicken Jardiniere**
1 medium grilled tomato
Iced tea with sugar substitute, if desired

DINNER

Cup of clear consomme (low-sodium if possible)
*Red Snapper Primavera**
2 medium boiled potatoes
½ cup broccoli
½ cup white wine diluted with seltzer water
2 peach halves in natural juices
Coffee or tea with sugar substitute, if desired

(6 glasses of water and calcium supplement per the Palm Beach Diet)

FRIDAY RECIPES

BREAST OF CHICKEN JARDINIERE

1½ teaspoons margarine
3 ounces boneless, skinless chicken breast
Pepper to taste
½ cup steamed carrots
½ cup steamed string beans
½ cup steamed cauliflower

Preheat sauté pan. Add 1 teaspoon margarine. Season chicken with pepper and place chicken in pan. Sauté each side, approximately 2 minutes per side.

Sauté vegetables with remaining ½ teaspoon margarine. Place vegetables on dinner plate segment by segment, and place chicken at center of plate. Lace with remaining pan juice.

RED SNAPPER PRIMAVERA

3 ounces red snapper
1 teaspoon whipped butter
Pepper to taste
Juice of ½ lemon
2 teaspoons white wine
½ teaspoon finely chopped parsley
½ teaspoon finely chopped dill
½ tomato, finely diced
½ clove garlic, minced
Pinch of oregano

Place red snapper in an ovenproof casserole pan greased with ½ teaspoon melted butter. Season with pepper. Combine rest of ingredients and place on top of snapper in casserole.

Place in oven and bake 10 minutes at 350° F. Remove from oven. Serve snapper with potato and broccoli; lace all with remaining pan juices.

SATURDAY

Calories: 1100–1200

BREAKFAST

¼ cup grapefruit juice
⅓ cup hot oatmeal sprinkled with 2 teaspoons raisins
¾ cup skim milk

MID-MORNING SNACK

¾ cup plain low-fat yogurt
2 low-salt crackers
Glass of water with twist of lemon

(Multivitamin/mineral supplement per the Palm Beach Diet)

LUNCH

Cup of clear broth (low-sodium if possible)
*California Salad**
Coffee or tea with sugar substitute, if desired

DINNER

Salad of Belgian endive
Dressing of 1 teaspoon lemon juice and 1 teaspoon salad oil
*Rack of Lamb Provençale**
1½ ounces Brie cheese
¼ pear

¼ apple
8 grapes
Coffee or tea with sugar substitute, if desired

(*6 glasses of water and calcium supplement per the Palm Beach Diet*)

SATURDAY RECIPES

CALIFORNIA SALAD

½ cup Bibb lettuce
⅓ cup watercress
⅓ cup avocado
⅓ cup raw spinach
1 kiwi, peeled and sliced
2 orange slices
2 grapefruit slices

Combine all ingredients and toss with lemon-oil dressing, made with 1 teaspoon of lemon juice and 1 teaspoon of salad oil. Sprinkle ½ teaspoon of raw slivered almonds over top, if desired.

RACK OF LAMB PROVENÇALE

SERVES 4

1½ pound rack of lamb (approximately 6 ounces per person)
1 teaspoon Dijon mustard
1 clove garlic, minced
1 teaspoon fines herbes
Pepper to taste
3 teaspoons bread crumbs
⅓ cup fresh or canned new peas
1 teaspoon chopped shallots

1½ teaspoons margarine
4 large tomatoes, hollowed out
1⅓ cups boiled broccoli stems
1⅓ cups boiled sliced carrots
1 teaspoon chopped parsley

Cut away excess fat from the rack of lamb, cleaning rib bones to the lean meat. Spread with the mustard. Season with garlic, fines herbes and pepper. Sprinkle with the bread crumbs. Roast in oven at 375 ° F for approximately 25 minutes.

Sauté new peas and shallots in half of the margarine. Fill hollowed out tomatoes with the peas and shallots. Place tomatoes in a sauté pan and bake at 375 ° F approximately 4 to 5 minutes—as the rack of lamb is finishing.

Meanwhile, sauté the precooked broccoli and carrots in the remaining ¾ teaspoon margarine. Ready 4 plates, and serve each person ⅓ cup broccoli, ⅓ cup carrots, and 2 3-ounce slices of lamb. Lace each plate with pan juices and garnish with a stuffed tomato and parsley.

SUNDAY

Calories: 1100–1200

BREAKFAST

½ grapefruit
1 slice whole wheat toast
½ teaspoon butter
Coffee or tea with sugar substitute, if desired

BRUNCH

*Chopped Sirloin Steak**
½ cup steamed julienne carrots
½ cup steamed Brussels sprouts
¾ cup strawberries
4 ounces dry champagne
Coffee or tea with sugar substitute, if desired

(*Multivitamin/mineral supplement per the Palm Beach Diet*)

DINNER

*Greek Salad**
*Shrimp Oreganato**
½ cup boiled rice
1 medium grilled tomato
⅓ cup boiled broccoli florets
4 ounces white wine diluted with seltzer water
½ cup sorbet or sherbet
Coffee or tea with sugar substitute, if desired

(*6 glasses of water and calcium supplement per the Palm Beach Diet*)

SUNDAY RECIPES

CHOPPED SIRLOIN STEAK

3 ounces chopped sirloin
1 tablespoon chopped parsley
½ cup fresh mushrooms
½ teaspoon margarine

Shape the chopped sirloin and parsley into a patty; set aside. In a nonstick skillet, lightly sauté mushrooms in the margarine; set mushrooms aside. Add sirloin patty to the skillet and cook to desired doneness, approximately 2–3 minutes each side. Serve mushrooms over the sirloin steak. Serve both with steamed julienne carrots and steamed Brussels sprouts.

GREEK SALAD

⅓ cup chopped iceberg lettuce
⅓ cup chicory
3 sprigs watercress
2 slices cucumber
2 slices tomato
5 small Greek olives
1 sliced radish
1 tablespoon finely chopped feta cheese

Combine all ingredients. Serve with a dressing of 1 teaspoon salad oil, 1 teaspoon red wine vinegar, a dash of oregano and a dash of lemon juice, mixed.

SHRIMP OREGANATO

5 large shrimp
2 teaspoons salad oil
2 teaspoons white wine
Juice of ½ lemon
1 clove garlic, minced
Dash of oregano
Pepper to taste
1 teaspoon margarine

Peel and devein shrimp and split in half lengthwise. Blend oil, wine, lemon juice, garlic, oregano, pepper and pour over shrimp. Heat margarine in a sauté pan, add shrimp with marinade, and cook 3–4 minutes. Serve shrimp with vegetables and rice; pour remaining pan juices over shrimp.

CHAPTER 10

Questions and Answers

You're sure to have a few questions about your diet now. Can you substitute foods? *Why* six glasses of water each day? What about the use of sugar substitutes? Your how-to-make-it-work queries are answered here.

Diet Questions

What if I "blow it" and go off the diet one day? Do I start the diet again the following day?

If you should slip up, get back on track at the next meal. Why wait for the following day? Listen, no one is perfectly self-controlled. Expect the occasional overindulgence. Accept it, start dieting again, and don't feel guilty about it. Life's too short to flog yourself with guilt over having enjoyed one slice of pizza.

Can I switch off one meal for another on the Palm Beach Diet? Can I have Wednesday's breakfast on Tuesday, for instance, and then Tuesday's breakfast on Wednesday?

Sorry, *no.* Each day of the Palm Beach Diet is nutritionally balanced. Therefore, each day should be regarded as an uninterruptable whole. Your meals are also ordered according to calorie content and hunger satisfaction. You won't find two light meals in a row, for example, or two heavy meals back-to-back. You're given an even diet pace. To begin to self-style the diet would jeopardize its effectiveness.

Another point: The weeks you spend on the Palm Beach Diet are your "training" for the *years* ahead. It will introduce you to new eating patterns and prepare you to *maintain* your slim new shape, once achieved. Follow it as is, and you'll learn to love satisfying yet nonfattening meals.

What if I really can't stand something on the diet? Can I make substitutions?

Allowed substitutions are indicated in parentheses in the diet meal plans. For example, you may substitute green peas for snow peas, or chicken for veal. An option generally is provided if the recommended item is either difficult to obtain or expensive.

If you absolutely refuse to eat something on the diet or are allergic to a particular food, you may substitute. See the list of foods in Chapter 12 for alternatives. Only make substitutions, however, as a last straw!

You'll note in the meal plans that you may substitute a commercially prepared frozen diet meal for one dinner and one lunch each week. For example, on the "core" week, you're allowed to have a frozen diet meal in place of Shrimp Scampi on Thursday night. If you choose the Shrimp Scampi, however, you may "save" the frozen diet meal, and have it in place of the entree on another night. In this way, if there is an entree on the diet you really can't bear, you have a ready substitute.

Remember, though, that a commercially prepared

frozen diet meal should not exceed 350 calories as a dinner replacement, or 300 calories as a lunch replacement. And of course, you may replace only one dinner and one lunch a week with a frozen diet meal.

If I choose to have a frozen diet meal once or twice a week, in place of the suggested entree, may I also have a salad or vegetables with it?

No. The frozen diet meal must substitute for the entire entree. If a dessert is part of the meal you're replacing with the frozen diet meal, you *may* still have the dessert.

If I cannot find a multivitamin/mineral supplement which exactly meets the recommendations spelled out in Chapter 7, what should I do?

As I mentioned earlier, vitamin/mineral supplements meeting these requirements are widely available. Perhaps you should try a larger supermarket or pharmacy. Don't worry if you find a brand which contains slightly more or less of these nutrients—so long as it contains each nutrient mentioned in *roughly* the recommended amounts. It is also perfectly fine and usual for multivitamin/mineral supplements to contain other nutrients along with those specifically cited on the Palm Beach Diet.

Should I choose a natural multivitamin/mineral supplement or are synthetic vitamins okay?

There is no difference between a natural and a synthetic vitamin. Each has the same chemical configuration and your body can't tell the difference. If you're asked to pay more for natural vitamins, choose a synthetic version instead!

I already take dolomite to supplement calcium in my diet. Can I continue to take dolomite, to the equivalent of 1000 mg. of calcium, rather than the antacid tablets you suggest?

No. Dolomite also may contain lead, arsenic, mercury and aluminum, which are dangerous. It's much smarter to get your calcium from food or from calcium supplements.

Are you seriously recommending antacid tablets as a way to get the calcium I need in my diet now?

Absolutely. Antacid tablets are far less expensive than most calcium supplements you can buy from vitamin and mineral manufacturers, or can get by prescription through your doctor.

To refresh your memory: You *only* want those antacid tablets which contain calcium carbonate and do *not* contain sodium or aluminum hydroxide. Excess sodium in the diet is unhealthy; aluminum hydroxide causes calcium to be liberated from bone, which potentially can weaken bone.

Taking five Tums or six Titralac each day will supply you with approximately 1000 mg. of calcium, which is roughly the supplemental amount you want now that you're fifty or more. You may take all of the tablets at once, chewing each in turn, or take them at various times during the day.

If you take antacids, remember to check with your doctor if you have kidney disease, kidney stones, a history of hypercalcemia (high blood calcium), drink a lot of milk, take vitamin D supplements or take calcium-blocking drugs. Also check if you use theophylline, a drug used for breathing disorders. Antacids can increase the potency of the drug. Antacids should not be taken with the drug cimetidine (Tagamet is the brand name) prescribed for ulcers and other stomach conditions; antacids can inactivate these drugs.

I hear that antacid tablets can cause constipation. Any truth?

Yes. The one possible disadvantage of calcium carbonate is constipation. The amount of calcium carbonate recommended here should not cause constipation in most people, however. And the generous intake of both fiber and liquids on this diet along with the recommended exercise will act as some insurance against constipation. If constipation is a problem while on the diet, however, try switching from the calcium carbonate antacid tablets to calcium *gluconate* supplements. They're available in most health food stores. You will have to take 5000 mg. of calcium gluconate, however—which will amount to a handful of pills. And calcium gluconate is relatively expensive. Nonetheless, for those few people for whom constipation persists, switching to calcium gluconate should provide relief.

The diet doesn't specify the amounts of some foods. For example, when tomato is called for in a sandwich, how much tomato can I have?

The diet assumes some common sense. In this case, a few slices of tomato—the amount you'd use to "build" a standard sandwich—is appropriate. When the diet calls for salad greens, for example, you may use a reasonable amount—half of a head of lettuce would be generous—roughly the amount you'd have in a big vegetable salad in a restaurant.

Where amounts are specified and measures provided, however, be strict. The first thing I ask my patients who report that they're not losing weight on the diet is the simple question: "Are your portions the correct size?" In many cases, they are not. Generally, overweight people are accustomed to eating big: They allow themselves too much meat, fish, poultry, rice, potatoes. It's easy to dish out twice the amount you need—or can have without gaining weight. Some dieters, too, are accustomed to weight-loss plans that allow, for example, all the protein foods—such as poultry and meat—that they can eat. This is *not* the case on the Palm Beach Diet; for medical and weight-loss reasons, we keep protein to a moderate level. Watch your portion sizes!

About amounts—when the diet calls for a piece of fresh fruit as a mid-morning snack, can I have any fruit? Can I have a whole watermelon?

Sorry, *no.* Choose an average-size piece of any medium-size fruit such as an apple or orange. You can have ½ to ¾ cup of berries such as strawberries and blueberries. Roughly a quarter of a melon is the right size; watermelon, a single-serving wedge. Fruit cocktail, fresh pineapple, etc.? About half a cup.

By the way, why am I allowed a mid-morning snack in the first place? Isn't that a peculiar time of day for a snack—seeing that I'm rarely hungry in the morning?

There's a metabolic reason for timing your calorie intake in this manner. Studies confirm that consuming a day's calories in many small meals is less "fattening" than consuming the day's calories in one or two large meals. Many dieters, for example, eat sparingly during the day and "save" their calories for a whopping evening meal. They would lose more weight, however, if they spread the evening meal's calories out during the day, eating smaller amounts at more regular intervals. Spacing meals is one small "trick" you can play on your metabolism, to save a few pounds a year!

Why does timing count in calorie-counting?

The body uses calories to digest and metabolize food. The more frequently you eat, the more energy the body uses in order to digest and "process" food. Of course, you can only lose weight in this manner by increasing the *frequency,* and *not the calorie content,* of your meals.

How you time eating and exercise can work to your weight-loss benefit, too. If you eat a large dinner and then go to bed for the night, you will gain more weight (or lose less) than if you eat and stay active for a period after the meal. Those unburned calories will be stored as fat! So, again, it's best to spread a day's calories throughout the day.

I like the idea, too, that you're receiving your multivitamin/mineral supplement mid-morning with a piece of fruit, which will contain some vitamin C. Vitamin C will encourage the absorption of iron in the supplement.

The diet calls for six glasses of water a day. It specifies either tap water, mineral water, seltzer water, or sparkling water. What about club soda? Is that allowed? It's low calorie.

You're right: Club soda is low-calorie. (Tonic water, meanwhile, can contain as many calories as soft drinks.) Most club sodas contain a lot of sodium, however. For this reason, I prefer that you avoid club soda.

Remember, too, that you can opt for a twelve-ounce can of diet soda, *maximum,* each day, in place of one glass of water. I don't *encourage* this, however; I prefer water to diet soda.

Black coffee and clear tea may *not* substitute for water.

Why am I asked to drink six glasses of water a day on the diet?

Among other things, in order to get rid of waste products from the body. The optimal amount of liquid per day is from eight to ten glasses. You get some liquids from food, of course, and from beverages other than water. The six glasses of water per day on the diet guarantee sufficient intake.

By the way, anyone on a diet will lose some water from the body. On the Palm Beach Diet, water loss is minimal, but deserves compensation. Water is essential to the functioning of all cells in the body.

When you recommend using salt substitutes "in moderation," what do you mean?

I mean it's best to "shake" the salt habit altogether! There's enough hidden salt in foods without adding more at the dinner table. If you insist on flavoring your food in this way, however, you may use a salt substitute sparingly—I mean one shake, or a few crystals, per meal. You need less of a salt substitute than you do salt to achieve the same salty taste.

Most salt substitutes contain potassium. Potassium is needed by the body to a point, but can be harmful in excess. Potassium intake should be restricted by those people with kidney trouble, and individuals who use certain kinds of diuretics. While most diuretics can deplete the body of potassium, and may require a potassium supplement, other diuretics don't affect the body's potassium levels at all. If you use a diuretic, and have any questions about use of salt substitutes, check with your doctor.

Speaking of sodium—what if package directions recommend using salt in cooking water: in vegetables and rice, for example.

Don't follow package directions regarding added salt. Your vegetables and rice can do without added salt. Do not use salt for cooking or for flavoring. If you must, use a small amount of salt substitute.

By the way, it's smart to compare labels for sodium content. You will find that some brands of cereals, for example, contain considerably more sodium than do other brands. Opt for the brand containing the least amount of sodium.

May I use sea salt in place of table salt?

No. There's little difference between sea salt and regular table salt in terms of its effect on your sodium intake. In fact, sea salt contains less iodine and it can be high in pollutants!

The diet calls for skim milk in coffee or tea. May I also use a nondairy creamer if I choose to?

Skim milk is a better choice. Many powdered nondairy creamers contain about 60 percent sugar! The liquid nondairy creamers generally contain sugar, in the form of corn syrup solids, and also may contain hydrogenated coconut oil or palm oil. The best choice among nondairy creamers are those made with polyunsaturated fat—but I still prefer that you use skim milk when possible. Of course, you also can take coffee or tea black.

I'm not allowed to use sugar. But can I use honey? Or raw sugar?

No. Honey is composed of glucose and fructose. It's chemically similar to table sugar. While refined sugar contains no nutrients, honey contains minuscule amounts of some nutrients—but you would have to consume ten cups of honey, for example, to meet your daily iron need. But honey and sugar add calories, and little else, to your diet.

Raw sugar is less refined than standard table sugar, but in this instance, "unrefined" doesn't bestow some sort of health benefit. It simply means that the sugar has been picked over for dirt and bugs! There are no health advantages to raw sugar. Avoid both.

Brown sugar, meanwhile, contains a small amount of calcium—but certainly not enough to warrant adding it to your diet. You would need to consume at least three cups of brown sugar to meet your daily calcium need.

May I use saccharin?

Be prudent. Saccharin, in quantity, may cause cancer. It also can increase your appetite.

What about sorbitol?

Sorbitol is a sugar—and contains as many calories as sugar—but it is absorbed more slowly by the body than sugar. That means it causes a less dramatic rise in blood sugar. It is used in a number of sugarless mints and sugarless gums: it carries the advantage over sugar of not being associated with tooth decay—but it can cause diarrhea if taken in excess amounts. Diabetics should *not* use sorbitol. Nondiabetics can use sorbitol on the Palm Beach Diet—in moderation.

What about NutraSweet and Equal?

NutraSweet and Equal are products containing *aspartame,* an amino acid-based sweetener. It's low-calorie and very sweet. It is allowed, in moderation, on the diet. Do not use excessive amounts of aspartame, however. The federal Food and Drug Administration is investigating reports of adverse reactions to aspartame when used in excessive amounts. Seizures, for example, were reported in one case where aspartame, and aspartame-containing soft drinks, were taken extensively on a daily basis. So be prudent—there are no reports of problems linked with normal use of aspartame.

It seems as though the term "sugar substitute" occurs in the diet meal plans several times every day. Why is this?

It does, but as an option only. You of course can have coffee or tea without a sugar substitute, too. If you choose to use one, use as little as possible per beverage.

Can I microwave my meals if I choose to?

Certainly. Microwaving, in fact, is the only cooking method which does not destroy vitamins. (No cooking method destroys minerals, which withstand heat admirably.) Feel free to adapt the recipes to your microwave oven.

"Steamed" vegetables are often specified on the diet. How do I steam vegetables properly?

You steam vegetables by keeping them raised above simmering water, so that the moist heat, and *not* contact with the water itself, does the cooking. Place the vegetables in a fold-out steaming rack, or in a wire-mesh strainer, and place it into a pot which contains one-half to one-inch of water. Cover the pot tightly, heat the water to a gentle boil and then cut the heat back to a simmer. The vegetables are done when they can be easily pierced with a fork. Remember to keep an eye on the pot: replace evaporated water if the water level becomes dangerously low. Do not oversteam.

I am surprised to see that coffee is allowed on this diet. Isn't it unhealthy for people over fifty?

Some people cannot tolerate coffee; it makes them nervous or depressed. This has to do with individual biochemistry, not age, however. If you enjoy coffee, there's no reason not to continue having up to two or three cups a day. This amount will not endanger the health of the majority of people. Over six cups a day, however, can cause nervousness and heartbeat irregularities. Keep yourself to three cups a day, maximum. Remember to use sugar substitutes in moderation, too.

What about special dietetic foods? Most are low in sodium and low in sugar. Can I use these canned foods in place of fresh?

Fresh is best. You don't really need special dietetic foods—and they tend to cost more than regular canned foods. Unless your doctor has prescribed them, to accompany a restricted sodium diet, for example, you can do without them.

What exactly do you mean by "whole grain bread?"

Whole grain bread has *not* been processed to the extent that nutrients have been compromised. It is slightly more expensive than white bread, "cracked wheat," etc., but worth the little extra. Breads which are "whole grain" or "whole wheat" say so on the packaging or wrapper.

The notation "natural," by the way, shouldn't influence you one way or the other. It doesn't mean a thing. For more on how to become a discriminating shopper, see Chapter 13, "More New-Age Survival Tactics."

What about diet candies?

Most contain calories. Some contain about twenty-five calories per piece. Eat enough of them and you'll gain weight! Go without.

Can I use those high-fiber wafers advertised as slimming aids? I want fiber in my diet, don't I? And I want to lose weight. Maybe I can kill two birds with one biscuit!

Appetite-reducing wafers generally contain cellulose—a fibrous substance which, when filled with water during digestion, helps fill the stomach. That gives you a full feeling—temporarily. These wafers won't help you lose weight in the long run, however. They don't affect the determinants of hunger—things like blood sugar levels and the amount of fat on the body. Your stomach may feel full, but your brain will still register hunger.

While you're on the Palm Beach Diet, and as you follow the weight-maintenance suggestions afterward, you will get plenty of fiber. You won't need additional fiber in the form of special wafers.

It's difficult for me to "swallow" the notion that I want carbohydrates in my diet. So many diet plans make a point of reducing carbohydrate intake.

The numbers speak for themselves. Carbohydrates contain four calories per gram. Protein also is four calories per gram—but most protein foods (such as meat, dairy products, poultry and fish) also contain fat, so you generally get about six calories per gram. Fat is nine calories per gram.

It's generally accepted, but incorrectly, that complex carbohydrate foods will make you fat fast! How many people, for instance, order a hamburger at a restaurant, remove the bun, and eat only the hamburger. They would consume fewer calories, in fact, if they had only half of the hamburger with the entire bun!

Where will I lose weight first? I seem to lose weight unevenly—from my face first, of all places.

There is no predicting where a person will lose weight. The tendency for women is to put weight on below the navel, and for men to put weight on above the navel. But in terms of losing weight, generalities are less accurate. Some people do seem to lose weight from their face first, while others lose more evenly from the whole body. Over the long term, you can expect to lose wherever you store fat—that only makes sense, of course. But saying what goes first, or faster, is impossible.

When I've dieted in the past, I came to rely on a quick restaurant lunch of a hamburger patty with a scoop of cottage cheese, and lettuce with tomato. Anything wrong with that?

That's basically good nutrition, but not optimal nutrition. This typical "diet plate" is higher in protein than necessary—especially if you plan to have meat, poultry or fish for dinner. Hamburger was "dissected" earlier in the book: It contains saturated fat, and much more phosphorus than calcium. Ideally, your diet should contain equal amounts of calcium and phosphorus. The cottage cheese *does* contain calcium—but less than many other cheeses. Cottage cheese also contains more sodium than many other cheeses. The lettuce and tomato? Terrific!

I don't see a "Chef's Salad" on the Palm Beach Diet. That's a diet staple, too, isn't it?

In my experience, people proceed to eat the meats and the cheese and leave the greens! Better-balanced, and lower in calories, would be a green salad containing fruits and vegetables with a little meat or a few nuts.

Another point: Salad dressings can be very high-calorie. Oils, mayonnaise and cream, remember, are fats. You can see how the combination of fatty cheeses and meats with a thick dressing—such as the creamy Italian "house" dressing served at many restaurants—can actually total more calories than a lunch of, say, fish, vegetable and potato!

Medical Questions

I'm "only" forty years old. Can I go on the Palm Beach Diet?

Certainly. Because it's safe for people over fifty, the Palm Beach Diet is safe for anyone. My only caveat is that premenopausal women be sure to get enough iron in their diet.

I'm surprised there aren't more health foods on the diet. I thought this was a health diet!

You may be suffering from some misconceptions about food and health. You'll want to read Chapter 13 closely. You're in for a few surprises.

I'm surprised at something else—no raw vegetables! Aren't carrot sticks, and raw vegetables for dipping, the ultimate diet-and-health foods?

They're terrific—unless you're old enough to remember that Wyle Post wore an eye patch!

With age, many people produce less gastric acid in the stomach; this inhibits the digestion of dense and chewy foods such as raw vegetables. Intestinal blockage can result. This danger is compounded if the raw vegetables aren't chewed well, due to sore gums, periodontal disease or dentures. Raw vegetables should not be a diet staple for elderly people or people with digestive or dental problems.

I've been taking enzyme tablets to help me better digest foods and absorb nutrients. Can I continue to take them on the Palm Beach Diet?

You can if you choose to waste your money. Hydrochloric acid in the stomach breaks down foods. This acid also inactivates enzymes as soon as they reach the stomach. The enzymes then are digested: They no longer exist! No way can they somehow aid in the digestion and absorption of food.

The pancreas makes digestive enzymes efficiently. You don't need to supplement unless you have a chronic pancreas condition.

The Palm Beach Diet supplies about 1000–1200 calories a day. But seeing that I'm taking a multivitamin/mineral supplement, can't I go on a lower-calorie diet and still remain healthy?

A lot of people think that a 500 calories-a-day diet is fine, as long as they're taking a fistful of vitamin pills to cover themselves against health problems. This is nonsense. Vitamins do not contain energy, *i.e.,* calories. They are substances without which certain body activities cannot take place—such as the building of bone or the formation of blood, but they cannot form blood themselves. You have to get energy for these processes from *food.*

There's no way you can lead a healthy life on a semi-starvation diet, because you must get energy. If necessary, the body will break down body tissue to do it.

What is the lowest calorie intake I can have each day without endangering my health?

Almost everyone will lose weight or at least not gain weight on 800 calories a day. To go below 800 calories a day for more than a few days is hazardous to your health. In fact, no one should take in fewer than 1000 calories a day without checking it out with their doctor first, *and* taking a multivitamin/mineral supplement while dieting.

My doctor has put me on a low-sodium diet. It allows no more than 2 g. of sodium each day. Can I go on the Palm Beach Diet?

Your doctor has put you on a severely sodium-restrictive diet. The Palm Beach Diet contains about 4–5 g. of sodium a day. If your doctor has you on less sodium, be sure to check with him or her before switching diets. Your doctor may veto your wish to follow the Palm Beach Diet.

If your doctor simply suggests that you "watch your sodium intake," however, you should be able to follow the Palm Beach Diet with your doctor's blessing.

I suffer from high blood pressure. Is the Palm Beach Diet safe for me?

This depends on the severity of your hypertension. Anyone on a sodium-restricted diet should check with his or her doctor before switching to this or any other diet. While the Palm Beach Diet can improve some cases of high blood pressure, it contains too much sodium (4–5 g. a day) for those on severe sodium restriction. *Most* people, however, require a certain amount of sodium for optimal kidney function: Severe restriction is not required.

Of course, any blood pressure medication should be continued during your diet. After you've lost weight, check with your doctor. He or she may find that your dose of blood pressure medication can be lowered.

My doctor has told me to reduce my cholesterol intake. Can I follow the Palm Beach Diet?

There are on average 200–300 mg. of cholesterol per day on the Palm Beach Diet. It should satisfy your doctor's low-cholesterol request—but do check first. He or she may advise you not to use butter, but to use margarine instead, for example.

Of course, if your doctor has prescribed cholesterol-lowering medication, or a special low-cholesterol diet, you must take his or her advice on the Palm Beach Diet. If you've been prescribed medication, do not go off it without your doctor's permission.

I take diuretic pills prescribed by my doctor. Will they interfere with the Palm Beach Diet—or vice versa?

Probably not—but it wouldn't be a bad idea to check with your doctor. Don't worry that you're bothering your doctor with a "silly" question. Doctors expect questions—and often are heartened that their patients are taking an intelligent interest in their own health.

I'm hypoglycemic. Can I follow the diet? Can a friend of mine who is diabetic?

A person who is hypoglycemic usually suffers from reactive low blood sugar. The Palm Beach Diet is compatible with this condition, and may very well help to stabilize it. I must add, though, that hypoglycemia is not as common as some people believe. Symptoms can be present without the condition itself being present.

The Palm Beach Diet is also a sound diet for people suffering from diabetes. In fact, it may reduce the symptoms or severity of mature-onset noninsulin-dependent diabetes. Get your doctor's okay, though, before switching diets.

I suffer from arthritis. How will the Palm Beach Diet affect it?

By losing weight you may notice some relief, but no diet can cure arthritis.

Can't certain foods help arthritis? I understand that vinegar, honey, lecithin, and cod liver oil can help relieve arthritis.

Sorry, there is no known nutritional antidote to the symptoms of arthritis. But that doesn't stop people from spending $25 on arthritis quackery for every $1 spent on arthritis research, according to the Arthritis Foundation.

If you're overweight, losing weight can help decrease the stress on arthritic weight-bearing joints, such as knees and hips. In this way, the Palm Beach Diet can supplement the medications and care prescribed by your doctor.

I take a medication known generically as verapamil. I understand it blocks the activity of calcium. Is it compatible with the Palm Beach Diet?

Verapamil is known under the brand names Calan and Isoptin. Another calcium-blocking drug is nifedipine: Procardia is its brand name. These drugs are often prescribed for heart conditions. I expect we'll see more of them prescribed in the future for other conditions, too, including high-blood pressure and migraine. They block the flow of calcium in certain cells of the body.

Prescribed doses of these drugs are not significant enough to affect calcium in your diet. Nor will dietary calcium interfere with the action of these drugs, to the best of our knowledge. There are no substantiated cases of interactions to date, according to the Drug Information Service, Gainesville, Florida. However, verapamil and nifedipine have only recently been put into wide use. Check with your doctor if you take calcium-blockers before changing your dietary routine.

I have an ulcer. Will this diet hurt me?

The practice of prescribing special diets for ulcers is pretty much kaput! A well-balanced diet that is comprised of several small meals is your best dietary approach. Avoid alcohol, smoking, caffeine, spices and anything that irritates your ulcer.

There now are excellent drugs available which help heal ulcers, by the way.

I hear that alcohol raises the levels of something called HDL cholesterol in the blood. This is supposed to be a good thing, because it helps protect the heart. Is that right?

That probably is what you read. But you got half the story. It's true that one or two drinks a day can raise blood levels of a particular kind of cholesterol, high-density lipoprotein cholesterol. This has been thought to be beneficial, because HDL cholesterol appears to help protect the heart. Drinkers loved reading this: They thought they had evidence that a drink or two acts as a health boost!

Now, however, we're finding that there are two types of HDL cholesterol. The one that alcohol raises is *not* the one that protects the heart. So much for justification!

Of course, doctors have known all along that more than a few drinks a day is health-hazardous, and even one drink can be health hazardous to someone with a drinking problem.

I've read that charcoal-broiling foods is unhealthy. What's the latest verdict?

Charcoal-broiled meats and fish have only been shown to cause cancer when chemicals which may be increased after charcoal broiling meat are applied in high concentrations for long periods of time to the skin of shaved mice! While there is concern in the medical community that charcoal broiling may produce cancer-causing substances, the evidence thus far is that the hazard to humans is minimal at best. Enjoy an occasional charcoal-broiled meal. Just don't overdo.

What about mercury in fish? There's a lot of fish on the Palm Beach Diet, for example.

Commercial sales of swordfish and tuna once were banned because of high mercury levels. Subsequent studies showed that the selenium in fish rendered the mercury harmless, however. The mercury level of fish caught off the U.S. coast has been watched by the Department of Agriculture carefully in recent years: No one has shown that there is a toxic level of mercury in fish.

Isn't carotene helpful in preventing cancer?

You may want to review the section on vitamin A in Chapter 4 (pp. 35–36). Carotene, a precursor of vitamin A, as well as vitamin A itself in other forms, can help prevent some cancers. Some people get carried away, however, and take carotene supplements in large doses. Carotene poisoning can result: It causes a yellow cast to the skin and can cause headaches. If you take carotene supplements and manifest either of these symptoms, stop taking the supplements. The symptoms will subside.

Are there good vitamins for sex? What about vitamin E? Or the mineral zinc?

There are no "sex vitamins." Vitamin E is vital to the development of secondary sex characteristics in rats, but it plays no such role in humans. Zinc allegedly is helpful in alleviating swollen prostate in men, but there is no evidence that it can help boost sexual prowess.

Which vitamins can give me quick energy, or help to reduce stress?

People like to think of vitamins as pick-me-ups. This notion doesn't jibe with the facts, however. The *fact* is that vitamins do not provide energy. Energy comes from calories, and there are no calories in vitamins.

The vitamin–stress connection is more complex. The deficiency of some vitamins can cause nervous reactions, but this generally occurs only when nutrients are severely imbalanced—in the case of alcoholism, for example, which depletes the body of B vitamins, and is often associated with a poor diet all around. When the body is stressed by such physical "events" as inadequate diet, illness or alcoholism, for example, there is an increased need for certain vitamins.

Your question, however, probably refers to such stress symptoms as nervousness, irritability, tension headache, diarrhea or constipation, and ulcer. Many health conditions can be aggravated or caused by emotional/chemical/physical distress. No vitamin can "erase" these symptoms, however, regardless of the claims made by manufacturers of "stress vitamins." If the telephone bill is due and you feel jumpy or if your boss is giving you a headache, a "stress vitamin" won't miraculously make it all better.

Of course, muscular tension, headache, ulcers, constipation and other stress-aggravated conditions should not be managed by popping a vitamin supplement and hoping for the best. Medical attention may be in order. And learning to deal with emotional challenges or problems without coming "unglued" is more effective than taking a "stress vitamin." I deal with stress in Chapter 15: Stress not only aggravates or precipitates health problems, it is a cause of overeating, too.

Can kelp speed up weight loss by speeding up the metabolism?

Kelp is a seaweed which contains iodine. Iodine is used by the body to make thyroid hormone; in turn, this hormone regulates the rate at which the body "works"—its metabolic rate, in other words.

This does not mean, however, that taking kelp can make a sluggish metabolic rate hop-to! Almost everyone gets sufficient iodine anyway. (The seafood-rich Palm Beach Diet is especially rich in iodine.) Getting *more* iodine does not make the thyroid produce *more* thyroid hormone.

Kelp is generally high in sodium, by the way.

Spirulina is from the sea, too, isn't it?

Yes. Spirulina are dried algae. Devotees maintain that they cure a list of health complaints that would fill the Dead Sea Scrolls! The substance is also touted as a reliever of hunger symptoms. Don't believe any of it! Apart from being a nice fiber source and containing small amounts of minerals and vitamins, spirulina is no big deal.

I've read that something called lecithin is helpful for weight-loss. What's the verdict?

You may also have read that it is helpful against heart disease, and helps to lower blood cholesterol levels. It has been promoted—in combination with kelp, vitamin B_6 and cider vinegar—as a weight-reduction aid.

Lecithin is a fat, derived from soybeans, egg yolk and corn. It's used in such diverse items as chocolate and cosmetic makeups as an emulsifier—that is, a substance capable of holding fat and water together.

Lecithin *cannot* help you lose weight; it does *not* help break down fats during digestion, as is claimed. It cannot help protect against heart disease, or lower blood cholesterol levels.

There *is* one health benefit that lecithin can bestow—but you would need to get such large amounts of it, you'd gain weight! Lecithin is a good source of choline. Choline has been shown to help improve memory: It is essential in the formation of brain neurotransmitters which control memory functions. You would have to get at least 5 g. of choline a day to *possibly* improve memory, however, according to laboratory studies. And to get 5 g. of choline a day, you would have to consume 30 g. of lecithin a day—an absurd amount, in other words. That would total about 400–625 calories a day in lecithin alone. And, because the effects of excessive amounts of lecithin are unknown, this would be an unwise practice indeed.

A friend of mine got HCG injections and lost weight!

HCG is human chorionic gonadotropin—a hormone extracted from the urine of pregnant women. The evidence indicates that it does *not* help in weight loss. HCG injections generally are accompanied by a 500 calorie-a-day diet. Your friend lost weight following the diet—not from the shots. And unsafely, I might add. A 500 calorie-a-day diet can be dangerous.

I take biotin—a B vitamin—for baldness. Is this practice compatible with the Palm Beach Diet?

Taking biotin for baldness is ineffective! Biotin does not restore hair in human beings. If a rat is deficient in biotin, it loses its hair. And if you put biotin back in the diet of balding mice, they regrow hair. Human beings do not lose hair because of biotin deficiency, however.

There is a new medication, incidentally, which is being tested as an antidote to baldness. The drug is called Minoxidil. Rubbed onto a bald area, it may regrow hair, seemingly without side effects. This drug, however, is years away from being made available. Until then, transplants—not biotin—is your recourse.

I'm realistic enough to realize that no diet can erase my turkey chin or baggy eyelids! I'm thinking about corrective surgery. Any thoughts?

Take care to find a competent plastic surgeon. And lose weight first, before having your facelift. I would suggest you reach and maintain your goal weight for several months, before surgery.

Can hair analysis determine what nutritional deficiencies I might be suffering from?

According to the Harvard Medical School Health Letter of March, 1984, hair analysis is "another way to get scalped." A number of laboratories do hair analysis to detect nutritional deficiencies. The main value of these tests is to detect high levels of toxic metals, such as arsenic. Otherwise, the results are generally unreliable. Two samples of hair from the same head, taken at the same time, can give two very different results. Factors which can skew the results include sweat, shampoo, beauty treatments, air pollution, rate of growth of hair and location on the head from which hair samples are drawn.

Besides, no one is sure that the levels of minerals found in the hair accurately reflect the levels of minerals in the body.

What do you have to say about chelation therapy, which I understand removes calcium from the blood stream so that it cannot contribute to hardening of the arteries.

Chelation therapy involves weeks to months of injections, at a cost of roughly $3000. Its purpose is to bind calcium and remove it from the bloodstream: By lowering blood calcium levels, goes the theory, calcium may be encouraged out of hardened plaques on artery walls, reducing their size. In turn, a reduction in plaque build-up would reduce the risk of cardiovascular disease.

Unfortunately, hardening of the arteries probably cannot be reversed in this manner. Plaques on artery walls, in fact, are made primarily of fibrous tissue, and not calcium. The chemical used in chelation therapy injections has not been shown to remove calcium. Once more, there is no evidence that the procedure helps prevent heart disease. Besides, you want to take, not remove, calcium!

I'm considering a procedure called liposuction, to remove fat from my thighs. Are you for or against it?

I'm still gathering information on this relatively new procedure, but I understand there can be problems with it. There are reports that the suction removal of fatty tissue from the thighs, for example, can result in irregular undulations of the overlying skin. A discrepancy in thigh circumference can result, with one thigh remaining larger than another. I wouldn't recommend committing to this procedure until more data is collected.

I'm considering jaw wiring to keep from overeating. Can you offer some advice on this procedure?

Don't do it! It's potentially dangerous. It's possible to aspirate the contents of the stomach and mouth into the lungs—and a doctor can't get at you quickly if your jaws are wired. This procedure also promotes gum and tooth disease.

CHAPTER 11

How to Pull It Off

It used to be called "will power." Will power was the stuff that you mustered to accomplish an arduous task—like dieting. Now psychologists talk about "behavioral modification"—a ten-dollar way of saying that you can be led to water *and* nudged into taking a sip or two. By changing the way you think about a diet and act when on a diet, you can increase your chances of diet success, in other words.

Anyone who has tried to lose weight can testify that will power alone is not much help. A puffed chest and gritted teeth rarely get the dieter over hurdles: The tendency is to fall for the first temptation. If people had to rely only on will power to lose weight, few pounds would be shed.

With the Palm Beach Diet, our focus is different. I won't lecture you on pluck and self-control. I'm not going to send you out cold to run some pretty tough hurdles on the strength of a pep talk! Instead, this chapter will *train* you for the event ahead—your diet, of course. It will prepare you for obstacles and weak moments.

I *will* ask you to *do* several things to help ensure diet success. These "nudges" will move you from the planning/plotting/day-dreaming stage to action. This game plan will give you a better chance of winning on your diet.

The Palm Beach Diet's 10 Success Strategies

I'm often surprised to see otherwise capable people fail to organize thier weight-control efforts. Ironically, *the very tools that assure diet success are the same strategies which build corporations, and underpin great achievements.* They are a group of simple yet elegant guidelines that have helped athletes run the three-minute mile; they've helped thousands of people overcome dependencies on alcohol or drugs. They will also help you lose weight.

1. Consider your timing.

It's generally best to start a diet when your life is relatively "quiet." If you have grandchildren coming to visit next week, it's no time to begin a diet. Your attention will be elsewhere. If you're in the middle of a demanding project at work, or are about to attend a three-day business conference, postpone dieting until next week. If you're an accountant, and it's the middle of tax season, start your diet on April 16! Dieting takes a certain amount of concentration at first, and there's no point in making your life more complicated than it has to be.

2. Set your goal.

Pin your diet goal to the mat. Perhaps you want to lose twenty pounds by a certain date. Maybe you want to wear once again a certain dress or evening jacket you "outgrew" several seasons ago. Perhaps your goal is to feel light enough to climb a particular flight of stairs you encounter—and shun—daily. Be specific about where you want to arrive—and when. Don't scattershot your efforts with vague longings such as "I want to lose weight" and "I want to feel better." Pinpoint a target. It will direct and motivate your efforts.

Some people find it helpful to contract with themselves to lose "X" number of pounds by a certain date. (The goal must be realistic, of course.) They draw up a written contract, and sign it—as a pledge to themselves. This is one certain way of affirming your commitment.

3. Easy does it!

Losing weight, like any major change in your life, is a process which involves psychological transformation, too. As you lose weight, your attitude toward losing weight will change! Slowly, it will become natural to look and to feel thinner.

This important psychological shift won't occur in a day or over a weekend, however. Just as any change—be it a new job or a new relationship—requires an adjustment period, adjusting to the fact, not the fantasy, of weight loss takes time. So easy does it. Remember: Too fast too soon doesn't last.

Be easy on yourself, too. If you should slip up and tuck into your nephew's birthday cake, don't brand yourself a failure. Don't even feel guilty about it. Guilt generally spurs dieters on to further bingeing, which creates more guilt, which results in yet more bingeing. A downward spiral is set in motion.

One goof isn't going to ruin your diet. If you slip up once or twice, accept it. You're human! Then mount your diet campaign again, at the next meal; forget the mistake happened. Want the truth? Guilt over a slip-up is more diet-destructive than the slip-up itself. Don't berate yourself; forget it and move on.

4. Take it one day at a time.

Making a major change in your eating habits is a tall order, but you don't have to do it all at once. Just do it one day at a time. Set your goal firmly in mind, and concentrate on today only. Forget tomorrow.

This is a key principle for an obvious yet often overlooked reason: Concentrate on the little things that need doing now, and the big things will follow automatically. Small and steady steps turn idle daydreams into wonderful reality.

Be prepared to go to any length to diet *just for today.* If it gets tough, chop the day into hours. Have a cup of tea and a few sugarless mints to get you through. Or make up a bowl of salad greens with low-calorie Palm Beach Dressing if you become really hungry. Anyone can stay on a diet for one day.

5. Enlist support.

There's strength and motivation in numbers. Corporations are united bodies of people working toward a common goal. Committees draw on the talent and the time of several people to achieve an end. In rehabilitation programs, working as a group is a keystone of success.

You may have heard this before, in your dieting past: Dieting with someone else is often a keen motivator. Having someone with whom you can share diet "notes" and general chit-chat helps hold your interest. Another person also acts as a sounding board for questions and complaints, and someone to share joys and accomplishments.

The buddy system works best, of course, if you and your dieting partner follow the same diet. If you can't find another willing (and ample!) body, however, nothing says you can't enlist the support of someone who *isn't* dieting. A friend who is a good listener will do nicely. You simply need someone you can talk to.

If you choose to diet with someone else, be warned that dieting duets can occasionally hit a sour note. How? Dieting with someone else can backfire if you team with someone who is not as committed to losing weight as you are.

A common scenario, for example, is this: You're a married woman who decides to diet. You read through the Palm Beach Diet and are heartened by its interesting menus and its medical soundness. It dawns on you that this is a diet plan that your husband could benefit from, and enjoy, too. He can have oatmeal, fettuccine, pancakes—real "man's food." At the same time, he can safeguard or improve his health. Bristling with good intentions, you coax him into joining you on the diet.

You might guess what happens next. Because you made this dieting decision for him, your husband isn't fully committed to your shared adventure: He's merely going along with the idea. And it's only a matter of time before he gives up the diet—which, in turn, disappoints you. Your disappointment may discourage *you* from continuing to diet.

Unless you find a diet partner as eager as you are, it may be smarter to enlist support from a nondieting friend or relative. Or you might reach a compromise with members of your family: You can ask them to join you in only the dinner portion of your diet. That frees them to eat whatever they choose the remainder of the day. It keeps the family dinner tradition intact, and it cuts down on cooking as well. The dieter isn't tempted by other calorie-laden entrees at the table, and non-dieters feel smug in the knowledge that they're watching their weight "part-time" and helping you get fit.

Enlist support, then—but find a dieting buddy who promises to be an asset.

6. Don't change the rules.

At this point in your life, you may be an old hand at dieting. If that's the case, I already can hear the wheels turning: "I'll omit this, and substitute that" or "I'll skip the mid-morning snack, and save it for after dinner."

Some of my patients, for instance, report to me that they like the Chicken Chutney Salad, or their morning oatmeal well enough, but they left the nuts *out.* "Too much bother," they say, with a dismissive wave of a hand. While they may have saved ten seconds, however, they've lost some calcium, zinc, fiber and protein. They've also omitted a bit of monounsaturated fat—the safest type of fat—which would have helped fill them up.

Another rationalization (dieters are expert at them): "I'll skip the mid-morning fruit and have it tonight for dessert. I'm not hungry mid-morning." And what happens? Because calories were skipped early in the day, hunger sets in later, in the evening. Visions of German chocolate cake start dancing in their heads.

The problem with reinventing the diet, then, is that you make mistakes. Most dieters *want* to be told what they can and cannot eat for this reason: They realize that, left to their whims, they'll skip the lima beans and have a loaf of garlic bread instead. Many dieters, at least temporarily, require the enforced discipline of meal plans carved in granite.

Rearranging the diet also can twist its nutritional and medical principles into pretzels! Remember that the Palm Beach Diet is deliberately and carefully balanced. Each day's meals have to be combined as given in order to maintain key nutrient and biochemical balances.

Fiddling with diet menus in this way reminds me of the dieter who, bursting with good intentions, went into a supermarket and bought all the groceries she would need for the first days of her diet. She toted her brown bags-full of groceries into the kitchen, and began loading items into cupboards and the refrigerator. Then curiosity, and habit, got the better of her. Here were foods she had never tried before—dates, nuts, pita bread, tropical fruits. So she started "testing" them all. She popped a few dates into her mouth. She liked them, which spurred her on to further experimentation. By the time she had put away the groceries for her new diet, she had consumed half a day's worth of calories.

Lesson learned. Don't nibble on a few crackers as you unpack your groceries, pledging to cut back on something else later in the day. A little unchecked snacking generally turns into *a lot* of extracurricular eating activity. Don't change the diet: It works as it stands.

7. Make pleasure an incentive.

People rarely follow through on a difficult task unless they derive some pleasure from it. So make a point of turning this into a pleasurable experience: At mealtimes, don't simply flop your food onto a plate, and plop *it* on the dining room table with a thud and an air of resignation. Enjoy the frills of fine china and flatware, candles and flowers. Play some music in the background. Make this an opportunity to pamper yourself. Make the process of dieting as attractive as the goal—and the goal moves that much closer to home.

8. Change old routines.

Here'a a big step toward diet success. Its lesson is obvious, but, once again, frequently overlooked. That lesson: If you've failed at something in the past, don't repeat the same mistakes again.

Do you always nibble at something in front of the television, after dinner? For the time being, read a book instead. Or better yet, watch television in a jogging suit—as a reminder that you're serious about getting into shape. Do some stretches in your chair or on the floor as you follow the television program.

Do you have a pastry everyday during coffee break? Make a point of stocking a desk drawer with sugarless mints—and bypass the pastry.

Have you shopped the same supermarket for years? Can you trace the steps to the bakery counter in your dreams? Switch markets.

The point of these exercises, of course, is to pull you out of ruts that encourage overeating.

Changing self-defeating routine is so important, in fact, that I'm going to ask you to shake up your eating habits two ways.

- Before you begin your diet, give your kitchen cupboards a thorough going-over. I don't mean with a cleanser and disinfectant. I mean with your eyes and your appetite! Identify, and then remove, food items that are not on the diet and may tempt you to stray. Toss them out, or give them to family or friends. Bags of cookies, boxes of cheese crackers, jars of dry roasted nuts are *out.* Anything that may beckon in a weak moment should be cleared out for at least the duration of your diet: Just spotting a box of those fancy cheese and garlic croutons in the cupboard may seduce you into an impromptu snack. Ensure—don't tempt—fate. Remove any food item you recognize as an incitement to nibble!

Search-and-destroy in your refrigerator and freezer, too. Frozen pizza? Out. The half-and-half you use in coffee? Give it to co-workers at the office. Peppermints you keep on hand for the neighbor's children? Offer them orange juice instead.

Of course, clearing tempting snacks from the kitchen may not meet the approval of other family members. Husbands or wives who aren't dieting may insist on keeping their snack food and beverages. If that's the case, ask them for a small favor. Your slightly unusual request: That they remove snack foods from the kitchen and keep them out of sight. *Hide* them, if necessary. By keeping nonperishable convenience foods out of sight, they remain out of mind (or at least out of reach!) to you, the dieter.

This request may sound extreme. It is, but if it will ensure you a diet "clean slate," then do it. It all but guarantees against absentminded or mischievous lapses.

This device also serves another purpose: It reminds you that eating is no longer a business-as-usual matter. You're breaking old routines and forming new habits. You're in a transition period, and transitions often require that you consciously "bury" old ways and practice new approaches.

As you divest your kitchen of diet-razing foods, remind yourself that you're not entering into new depths of deprivation! This measure simply safeguards against *over*eating.

• Bear with me on this one, because it is something diet plans generally don't ask of you. At first, this request may seem outside the scope of the diet; it may seem irrelevant to weight loss. It *is* pertinent and rooted in psychological fact, however. I call it the "pleasure displacement principle."

Psychologists know, for example, that when a person is deprived of a pleasurable habit, they sometimes experience a painful loss. A void is created—a void that needs refilling. That sense of loss can be eased if replaced with something equally pleasing.

Now that you've forfeited the pleasure of snacking, you will want to replace it with another pleasure. You want to divert the time and the energy you spent on food into another channel.

So divert it! Start a project or indulge a new interest at the time you begin to diet. Make it something you've always wanted to do, but have never gotten around to. Make it something that promises to really turn you on. Perhaps it's starting a videotape library. Maybe it's making a point of playing a golf course in each of the fifty states. Plan a trip to your home country—or home state, for that matter. Whatever you choose to do, make it something happy—and distracting!

9. HALT!

What is HALT? It's an acronym for a phrase used in rehabilitation programs: "Don't let yourself get *h*ungry, *a*ngry, *l*onely or *t*ired."

When you're hungry, your defenses are down. You enter into a pitched battle with yourself: Should I or shouldn't I? Don't play the hero or heroine. Don't try to ride out a sensation of hunger. Instead, make a cup of tea and have a few sugarless mints.

For some people, overeating is a way to vent inner emotional "steam." Bingeing often is the explosive and self-destructive release of suppressed feelings. How much healthier, though, to express those feelings openly—rather than in the surreptitious glow of the refrigerator light bulb at one o'clock in the morning.

How? If it's anger that prompts you to overeat, try to talk it out with the person who upset you. If that's not possible, get a punching bag! Or throw shells into the ocean. Slap great stretches of paint on canvas. Whatever you do, don't take your anger out on yourself. Release and relieve it in an appropriate, harmless way.

Loneliness is another spur to overeating. Overweight people sometimes are lonely people, for whom food fills the "people gap." A vicious pattern can become routine: Lonely people may overeat, then feel guilty and even *more* set apart from others. That emptiness then leads to further bingeing.

This self-defeating pattern can be changed, however. People who feel they are struggling alone with a weight problem need to know they are *not* alone. Many other people experience these same feelings. How about asking a neighbor over for coffee? Or join a group or club . . . or get a pet?

Feeling tired, too, can deflate your motivation and enthusiasm. When you're tired, it's easy to justify a snack as a quick "pick me up." On the other hand, you can better resist old eating habits when you feel relaxed and rested. Make a point of getting plenty of rest while you're dieting.

10. Rise above poor excuses.

Walk down most corridors of achievement, and the last thing you'll trip over is a lame excuse, or a whine, or an "I would have, but . . ." In the first chapter of this book, we overturned dieters' excuses. Now, let's overturn some others.

THE EXCUSE	HOW TO ATTACK THE EXCUSE
"The diet's too hard."	Baloney. Not this diet. It's realistic and manageable. It's as hunger-proof as

THE EXCUSE	HOW TO ATTACK THE EXCUSE
	possible. Do it one day at a time—and you can make it very enjoyable. Refer back to points 3 and 7.
"The diet's too expensive."	Meat is more expensive than vegetables; snack foods are more expensive than most foods. Alternatives to expensive items are provided. Concentrate on "Easy Week"—the most cost-conscious of the three weeks. Remember that doctors' bills are *very* expensive; so think how much you can save in the long run.
"Too much preparation time."	Less preparation time than almost any healthy diet circulating now. You *could* live on fast foods, but how long or how well would you live?
"I *like* junk food."	But you don't enjoy being fatigued, ill or bored. Junk food generally is fattening; junk food is frumpy

THE EXCUSE	HOW TO ATTACK THE EXCUSE
	too: Whatever happened to aging—and eating—gracefully?
"My spouse eats more, and I have to watch!"	Don't watch. Get up from the table or your chair. Or stay put and realize there's more to life than an uneaten French fry on someone else's plate. Discuss your new project . . . or next summer's vacation. Hold your diet goal firmly in mind, and imagine yourself in clothes two sizes smaller.
"Food is a comfort."	Call a friend instead. Get active in a church group. Take a hot bath. Curl up snugly with an inspirational book. How about some part-time work—paid or volunteer? Find enjoyment and self-reliance in the project you're about to start.
"I eat when I'm angry."	Angry at someone or something else? Don't take it out on yourself. Why

THE EXCUSE	HOW TO ATTACK THE EXCUSE
	turn your anger inward? Get anger out of your system. Angry at yourself—for slipping up on your diet? Forgive yourself. Forget guilt. Start again today, and take it one step at a time.
"We all die sometime . . ."	But it needn't be prematurely, from a preventable illness.

PART THREE

Health Ammunition for the Mature Years

CHAPTER 12

How to Keep It Off

Let's gaze ahead for a moment. Several months have passed. Perhaps it's midsummer, and you've achieved your diet goal. Or it's midwinter, and you're able to ease into a suit that, last year, was tighter than a Miami accountant. You're thrilled, of course—and yet slightly disbelieving. At this point, it's natural to stop pinching yourself, and worry that your *wardrobe* will start to pinch you again. . .

"Weight rebound" is a post-diet peril. As I mentioned earlier, the main cause of weight rebound after dieting is overeating. And by "overeating," I mean choosing fattening foods again, in portions that would satisfy a small battalion.

I can hear you now: "But I can't help myself. In the past, whenever I was hungry, I'd reach for a candy bar or ice cream, and my appetite was appeased instantly. Now that I've lost weight, I *know* I can't have quantities of these foods without regaining weight. But I doubt I can stop myself. Having an apple just isn't the same thing when you're really hungry—and yogurt *does not* taste like sour cream."

Here's where you and I can share a secret. *Recent re-*

search demonstrates that certain types of nonfattening foods satisfy hunger cravings as fully as do fattening foods.

It amazes me at dinner parties and in restaurants to see people choose foods likely to go straight to their hips or stomach! Especially when they could pick foods which are just as filling, but not as fattening. They choose high-calorie foods, knowing that the creamed potatoes, or pizza or chocolate cake will fill them up and satisfy their taste buds. They assume that only fatty foods will satisfy their appetite. That's where they're wrong: We now know that calories and satiety are *not* synonymous. We also know that food preferences are learned, and that new food preferences can be learned and enjoyed.

Let me give you an example. A research project at the University of Alabama compared two meals for appetite satisfaction: One was high in calories—roast beef, creamed potatoes, green bean casserole and chocolate cake; the second meal consisted of less-fattening foods—chicken, brown rice, broccoli, whole wheat rolls and fruit. The first meal "weighed in" at 3000 calories; the second, at only 1570 calories. Surprise: Both obese and nonobese subjects found the lower-calorie meal as satisfying and enjoyable as the first.

Impossible? No, simple. The lower-calorie meal contained the higher-fiber, bulky sorts of foods called *complex carbohydrates.* Foods high in complex carbohydrates include whole grain breads and cereals, starches such as rice and potatoes, vegetables and fruit. The health benefits of complex carbohydrates are praised throughout this book: A few can help lower cholesterol levels, for instance; some can help prevent constipation, and reduce the risk of colon cancer; they're generally far more nutrient-rich than other foods, too. And now we find that these same health-supportive foods can fill you up without fattening you up! Now that's a discovery!

Complex carbohydrates satisfy in two ways. One: It takes longer to eat them than it does many high-fat or sweet foods. They're fibrous and dense foods, for the most part. In the Alabama study, it took 33 percent more time to consume the low-calorie meal than it did the high-calorie assembly. By literally having to chew and digest more food, it gives you time to feel full—even though fat and calorie content is lower.

Whole grains, starches, vegetables and fruits also stay in the stomach for long periods of time. This is one reason that a slice of bread satisfies you longer than one ounce of chocolate—even though both have roughly the same calorie count. True, *fat* and protein remain in the stomach even longer than complex carbohydrates, but complex carbohydrates are metabolic marathoners, too.

How do you apply this knowledge, then? In the future, when you're hungry, have a slice of whole grain bread or a few unsalted crackers instead of candy. If you find that one apple doesn't tame your hunger craving, have two.

Of course, the whole point here is that you shouldn't crave snacks if you use complex carbohydrates to make *meals* satisfying. I'll show you how.

Staying Thin ad infinitum

Now that you're off your diet, you don't want to become attached at the hip to a calorie counter, or have to weigh every morsel you put in your mouth. Both prospects are about as exciting as having to empty the trash!

Being chained to rigid meal plans isn't enticing, either. Many weight-loss plans provide the post-dieter with a maintenance diet that dictates the composition of every meal. The idea is to discourage weight gain by eliminating choice. Maintenance diets work only to the extent that they're followed doggedly and indeterminably.

I prefer a freer approach to weight maintenance, one that moves the dieter beyond props and gimmicks. An approach that lets you weight-watch "by ear"—recognizing foods and food portions you can "get away with" and remain healthy and trim.

To this end, I've compiled an honor roll of foods. Most combine assets—terrific nutrition, and hunger satisfaction, for example. Some are especially high in nutrients vital to the mature system. Some have a medical leg up on other foods—providing high fiber content, for instance. Others keep the biochemical balances I described earlier—they are basically low in sodium, high in potassium and moderate in phosphorus. A few of these foods have unique qualities: Almonds, for example, contain salicylate, a chemical cousin to the active ingredient in aspirin; about six raw almonds are the equivalent of one aspirin in pain-relief potential. Still others of these foods are simply—and deliciously—low calorie.

These, then, are the foods with which you can live happily (and thinly) ever after. Stock up on them!

THE PALM BEACH HONOR ROLL OF FOODS

GRAINS	CALORIES	PLUSES
Bran bread and cereals	105 calories/cup bran flakes 105 calories/ bran muffin	A complex carbohydrate and the best source of dietary fiber. High in potassium, magnesium, zinc, B vitamins, vitamin E. Beware sodium and sugar content of bran cereals: Read labels.
Brown rice	77 calories/⅓ cup, cooked	Superb complex carbohydrate: filling, yet not excessively calorie-high. Good source of iron and magnesium. 3–4 times the dietary fiber of white rice; 2–3 times the zinc and potassium; 5 times the vitamin E of refined rice.

(*continued*)

GRAINS	CALORIES	PLUSES
Oatmeal bread and cereals	200 calories/1½ oz. oatmeal	Good and inexpensive protein. High in fiber; decent iron source. Good source of potassium, magnesium and B vitamins.
Pasta	190 calories/cup spaghetti, cooked	Like the foods above, an appetite appeaser. Keep serving size, though, to 2–3 dry oz. Whole wheat, green (spinach and artichoke), and reduced calorie versions preferred. A good source of fiber, B vitamins, iron.
Shredded wheat cereal	90 calories/biscuit	Lower in calories and sodium than many commercially prepared cereals.
Whole wheat bread	65 calories/slice	Superb complex carbohydrate. Standout source of fiber. Contains nutrients removed from white bread—e.g., zinc, chromium, magnesium. Same calorie content as white bread.

VEGETABLES AND LEGUMES	CALORIES	PLUSES
Alfalfa sprouts	27 calories/cup	One of the few nondairy foods to contain more calcium than phosphorus. A good fiber source, and very low-calorie. Two preliminary studies (one in rats; the other in rabbits) found alfalfa inhibited cholesterol absorption.
Artichokes	15 calories/3 oz.	Very good source of potassium—which balances artichoke's sodium content. Good source of the B vitamin biotin. Satisfying. Often a substitute for potato or rice in Palm Beach—and less fattening than either.
Asparagus	30 calories/cup	Like artichoke, low in sodium and a potassium "star." High in vitamins A and C; good fiber. Surprisingly low calorie.
Bean sprouts	35 calories/cup	Low calorie; an okay source of fiber and iron in the bargain.
Belgian endive	10 calories/cup	Good source of carotene, folic acid, vitamin C, potassium. Reasonable source of iron. Very low in calories. Expensive, though.

(*continued*)

VEGETABLES AND LEGUMES	CALORIES	PLUSES
Broccoli	40 calories/cup	A vegetable of the Brassilica, or cabbage, family; regular consumption associated with reduced risk of some cancers. High in potassium, vitamins A and C, iron, folic acid, magnesium. Good fiber. Widely available at a relatively low cost.
Brussels sprouts	55 calories/cup	A vegetable of the Brassilica family; regular consumption associated with reduced risk of some cancers. A good source of potassium, vitamins A and C, folic acid. A fiber source.
Cabbage	30 calories/cup	A vegetable of the Brassilica family; regular consumption associated with reduced risk of some cancers. Good fiber source. High in vitamins A and C; folic acid. Inexpensive and widely available.
Carrots	50 calories/cup	Great source of two important health/diet nutrients—potassium and vitamin A. Vitamin A bioavailability increases with cooking. A relatively high-calorie vegetable, however. Inexpensive and widely available.
Cauliflower	30 calories/cup	Another Brassilica family vegetable associated with reduced risk of some cancers. High in vitamin C, folic acid, and biotin—a B vitamin. Decent fiber source.
Chick peas	85 calories/2 oz.	Good source of fiber, protein, calcium, magnesium, iron. Significant source of sodium, however.
Cucumber	15 calories/8 slices	Main component: water. Good potassium (sodium-balancer) source.
Garlic	4 calories/clove	In large quantities, seems to raise the levels of heart-protective HDL cholesterol. Terrific flavor stand-in for salt. No restaurant in Palm Beach would be without!
Green beans	30 calories/cup	Top-notch diet veg.: only 15 calories per ½ cup serving. High in potassium, magnesium, vitamin A, folic acid. Like

(continued)

VEGETABLES AND LEGUMES	CALORIES	PLUSES
		cucumber, low in sodium, too. Decent fiber. Opt for fresh or frozen over canned.
Green and red pepper	15 calories/pod	Main component: water. Nice levels of potassium, vitamins A and C. Not as fibrous as green beans, however.
Leek	14 calories/2 oz.	Like onion, a good low-calorie source of fiber, potassium, vitamins A and C, folic acid.
Lentils	50 calories/2 oz.	High-ish calorie count, but a good protein and fiber source. High in potassium, magnesium, iron, zinc, niacin, folic acid and pantothenic acid, too. We found a popular brand lentil soup with celery and spinach for 79¢!
Lettuce greens	10 calories/cup	Very low calorie, and good source of fiber, potassium, vitamins A and C, folic acid.
Lima beans	190 calories/cup	Good source of potassium, iron, fiber, niacin. Relatively high in calories, though. Frozen lima beans generally contain some sodium, incurred during processing.
Mushrooms	20 calories/cup	Surprisingly good source of fiber: 10 small mushrooms have 8 times the fiber of ½ cup cooked macaroni. Good source of potassium, niacin, pantothenic acid—at a low-calorie cost. Some iron. Beware sodium content of canned mushrooms.
Onion	60 calories/cup	In large quantities, may reduce cholesterol levels. An excellent flavor-enhancer, and good source of vitamin C and potassium.
Parsley	1 calorie/tablespoon	A nutrient knockout. Splendid source of vitamin A. Standout source of vitamin C, and high in potassium, calcium, magnesium, iron, niacin and vitamin E. Fresh is much more nutrient-rich than is dried and flaked. Chop and use liberally in recipes.
Parsnip	100 calories/cup	Good source of potassium, vitamin C and folic acid. Very low in sodium.

(*continued*)

VEGETABLES AND LEGUMES	CALORIES	PLUSES
Peas, frozen	110 calories/cup	Nutrient-high, filling—but also higher-calorie than most vegetables. Keep serving sizes to ½ cup. Strong in potassium, magnesium, iron, vitamins A and C, niacin, folic acid. Sodium levels may be high in canned peas, moderate in frozen.
Potato	125 calories/ potato	It's not the calories in the potato, but the butter or sour cream you dollop on top that's the diet-razer. Good source of potassium, magnesium, niacin, vitamin C. (Retain vitamin C by cooking potato whole in its skin.)
Radish	5 calories/4 radishes	Low calorie, and a good source of potassium, vitamin C and folic acid.
Spinach	15 calories/ cup, raw 40 calories/ cup, cooked	A nutrient all-rounder. Contains calcium, iron and fiber—all terrific for the 50-plus years. Relatively high in sodium, yet high in potassium, too—the balance is fine. In addition: vitamins A and C, magnesium, folic acid. Low-calorie, low-cost.
Squash	30 calories/cup summer squash 130 calories/cup winter squash	Zucchini and summer squash low calorie. Winter and butternut varieties high in calories, but richer in nutrients, too. Nutrients, generally: vitamin A and potassium. Butternut squash a soaring source of potassium. Squash contains significant sodium, but generally offset by high potassium content.
Sweet potato	170 calories/ potato	Contains more vitamin A and E than white potato. Good fiber. Inexpensive. Higher in calories, though, than white potato.
Tomato	25 calories/ tomato	Actually a fruit, but considered a vegetable by many. High in potassium, vitamins A and C, biotin. Flavorful and useful.
Watercress	10 calories/2 oz.	Expensive, generally, but nutrient-rich. The line-up: calcium, iron, vitamins A and C, folic acid. Decent fiber. A diet and health bonanza similar to parsley and spinach.

NUTS AND DRIED FRUITS	CALORIES	PLUSES
Almonds, raw	6 calories/ almond	A Palm Beach favorite. Lower in fat (although still significant) and sodium than most nuts. Good source of potassium, magnesium, fiber, zinc, vitamin E, niacin, folic acid and protein. Excellent nondairy source of calcium. Almonds contain salicylates—a relative of the active ingredient in aspirin. About 6 raw almonds are the pain relief equivalent of one aspirin, according to a Harvard professor.
Cashews, raw	6 calories/ cashew	Lower in fat (although still significant) and sodium than most nuts. A source of iron, vitamin A, folic acid and protein. Higher in phosphorus and lower in calcium than almonds, however.
Dates	22 calories/date	A popular Palm Beach garnish that's high in potassium, magnesium and niacin. Good source of iron. A little goes a long way: relatively calorie-high.
Raisins	80 calories/oz.	Very good source of iron. High in potassium and magnesium as well. (Potassium, remember, balances sodium in the diet.) Inexpensive and widely available.

FRUITS	CALORIES	PLUSES
Apple	80 calories/ apple	High in potassium, and the peel is a good fiber source. The meat contains pectin, a fiber which, in quantity, reduces cholesterol levels. Inexpensive and widely available.
Apricot	55 calories/3 apricots 18 calories/ dried apricot	Very high in fiber. Good potassium, iron, vitamin A and magnesium.
Banana	100 calories/ banana	High in potassium and vitamin B_6. Good fiber source. Good magnesium, vitamins A and C. A high-calorie fruit, however: Use sparingly.
Cantaloupe	80 calories/½ cup	Potassium—again! Also high in vitamins A and C, and folic acid. Low-calorie.

(*continued*)

FRUITS	CALORIES	PLUSES
Cherries	45 calories/10 cherries	Good potassium. Very low in sodium.
Grapefruit	50 calories/½ grapefruit	A very good source of potassium. High in vitamin C. The white membrane an okay fiber source. Low-calorie and widely available.
Grapes	35 calories/10 grapes	Good potassium. Very low in sodium.
Honeydew melon	50 calories/ average wedge	Low calorie and decent source of potassium, vitamin C, folic acid.
Lemon	60 calories/cup lemon juice	The juice contains roughly the same amount of vitamin C as orange juice and grapefruit juice. A sublime flavor-enhancer. Serve lemon wedges with fish entrees and in tall glasses of cooled mineral, seltzer or spring water.
Lime	65 calories/cup lime juice	Not quite as high in vitamin C as lemon, but still a good source. Serve wedges with cantaloupe and serve in tall glasses of cooled mineral, seltzer or spring water.
Mango	55 calories/cup	Middle-of-the-road fruit in calories. Contains potassium, vitamins A and C—all health bonanzas for those 50-plus.
Orange	65 calories/ orange	Very good vitamin C and potassium source. Very low in sodium.
Papaya	55 calories/ papaya	Similar to mango.
Pineapple	80 calories/cup	Slightly lower calorie than mango and papaya. Lower in potassium, too.
Prunes	260 calories/cup	Watch calories—½ cup serving recommended. Very good fiber source. Contains some vitamin A. Noted for laxative effect.
Raspberries	70 calories/cup	Low calorie. Good potassium. Low sodium. Higher in fiber, ounce for ounce, than strawberries. About twice the calcium and magnesium of strawberries, too.

(*continued*)

FRUITS	CALORIES	PLUSES
Strawberries	55 calories/cup	Low calorie. Good potassium. Low sodium. A very good vitamin C source.
Tangerine	40 calories/tangerine	Similar to orange, but with significantly less vitamin C and biotin.
Watermelon	12 calories/4 oz. (with rind)	Main component: water. One of the lowest calorie fruits. Contains some potassium and pantothenic acid.

DAIRY PRODUCTS	CALORIES	PLUSES
Skim milk	85 calories/cup 100 calories/cup 1% low-fat milk 120 calories/cup 2% low-fat milk	Roughly half the calories of whole milk. With fat removed, relative protein content is higher, too. Same nutrient profile as whole milk: calcium, potassium, biotin, zinc, magnesium, vitamin B_{12} and pantothenic acid. Enriched skim milk also contains vitamins A and D. Contains sodium, too, however: Individuals on a sodium-restricted diet should check with their doctor regarding use of dairy products.
American cheese	95 calories/oz.	Lower in fat than cheddar. Lower in calcium and vitamin A, though, than cheddar.
Cheddar cheese	115 calories/oz.	Very good calcium source. High, too, in potassium, zinc, vitamins A and B_{12}, niacin. Good protein source.
Cottage cheese	165 calories/cup 1% low-fat 205 calories/cup 2% low-fat	Low-calorie, and good source of protein. Pretty decent calcium. Higher in sodium than many other cheeses, however.
Edam cheese	101 calories/oz.	Lower calorie count than cheddar cheese, but still significantly calorie-high: Be judicious. High in potassium and sodium, and lower in vitamin A, than cheddar. As is true of all cheese: a good protein and calcium source.
Mozzarella	85 calories/oz.	Similar to Edam; a bit lower in calories.
Low-fat yogurt	145 calories/ 8 oz.-tub plain	Good source of calcium, potassium, niacin. Fairly high calorie, though.

(*continued*)

DAIRY PRODUCTS	CALORIES	PLUSES
	230 calories/ 8 oz.-tub fruit-flavored	Choose low-fat plain, or those flavored with coffee, lemon or vanilla. Yogurts containing fruit are generally high in sugar.

FISH AND SEAFOOD	CALORIES	PLUSES
Bass	Not available	While exact calorie values for bass are not available, it is considered a middle-of-the-road fish in terms of calories. Darker fish generally is higher-calorie than white fish. Good protein source. Good niacin.
Bluefish	135 calories/3 oz. (baked with butter or margarine)	A darker fish, higher in calories and fat than white fish. Higher in cholesterol than white fish and many meats. However, high polyunsaturated-fat level helps reduce blood cholesterol levels. A good source of protein, potassium, niacin, vitamin B_{12} and biotin.
Clams	65 calories/3 oz. (raw, without shells)	Low fat and good protein. Good source of iron, vitamin A, biotin and potassium. Clams have a 3:1 ratio of phosphorus to calcium, however.
Cod	70 calories/3 oz. (with bones and skin)	Like all white fish, a terrific low-calorie source of protein. Cod is marginally better in fat profile than sole, for example, containing a little less cholesterol and more polyunsaturated fat, which helps reduce blood cholesterol levels. White fish contains monounsaturated fats, too—the "neutral" and safe fat. Nutrient rundown: Sodium and potassium are balanced. A good source of niacin and biotin.
Crabmeat	135 calories/cup	Good protein, iron and magnesium. Fairly low-calorie. Be judicious, however: Crabmeat is fairly high in cholesterol compared with other fish; sodium outranks potassium. Shrimp and lobster are worse offenders, however.

(*continued*)

FISH AND SEAFOOD	CALORIES	PLUSES
Flounder	Not available	See cod.
Grouper	Not available	See cod.
Halibut	85 calories/3 oz. (with bones and skin)	See cod.
Mackerel	118 calories/3 oz.	See bluefish.
Mussels	75 calories/3 oz. (without shells)	High protein; low fat; good calcium, iron, zinc and niacin. However, like most seafoods, sodium swamps potassium levels. Cholesterol levels are significant, too. White fish a better health bet, generally.
Oysters	160 calories/5 medium	Low fat, good protein, and high in calcium, iron, copper, zinc. Terrific source of vitamin B_{12}. Contain about half the cholesterol of mussels; lower in cholesterol than most fish, meat and poultry. Good source of vitamin A, niacin and biotin. Watch sodium level, however.
Pompano	Not available	See bluefish.
Salmon	169 calories/ 3 oz.	Good protein. Good source of pantothenic acid and biotin.
Scallops	90 calories/ 3 oz.	Like cod and oysters, a seafood "of choice." One of the lowest levels of cholesterol among seafood. A good potassium to sodium ratio—although higher in sodium than potassium. Good source of protein, calcium, niacin. An okay source of iron.
Sole	55 calories/3 oz. (with bone and skin)	See cod.
Swordfish	Not available	Good protein. Very good source of vitamin A. Contains a bit of iron, too. Contrary to popular belief, swordfish is low in fat. A Palm Beach favorite—although not readily available throughout the country.

(*continued*)

FISH AND SEAFOOD	CALORIES	PLUSES
Trout	76 calories/3 oz. (with bone and skin)	Similar to bluefish. Contains more cholesterol than cod, but not as much as sole.
Tuna, water-packed	117 calories/3¼ oz. can	Not particularly low-calorie as seafood goes: similar to poultry in calorie count. And higher in sodium than potassium—a 2:1 ratio. But a good and widely available source of protein, zinc, niacin, the B vitamins and vitamin D.

POULTRY	CALORIES	PLUSES
Chicken	120 calories/3 oz. (light meat)	Poultry generally is lower in sodium than fish. It tends to be higher in calories than white fish; lower in calories than dark fish. Remove the skin, and you remove most of the fat—a good practice, indeed. For nutrient profile, see turkey.
Turkey	114 calories/3 oz. (light meat)	Poultry rule of thumb: Dark meat contains more cholesterol than white meat. Turkey is a "sleeper": It gains on chicken several ways. It contains fewer calories and a bit more protein ounce for ounce. Turkey contains half of the fat of skinless chicken! And it contains only ⅔ of the sodium of chicken. Both contain potassium, calcium, magnesium, phosphorus and iron, plus niacin, biotin and pantothenic acid. Turkey has 1½ times the zinc of chicken.

MEATS	CALORIES	PLUSES
Lean beef	222 calories/3 oz. sirloin	Calorie values of meat are difficult to assess because they vary significantly cut to cut. Good protein and excellent iron source. Also high in zinc, niacin, vitamin B_{12}. Beef has the lowest sodium content of all meats. On the down side: contains many times more phosphorus than calcium. And meat fat is saturated fat, the unhealthiest sort.

(*continued*)

MEATS	CALORIES	PLUSES
Lean lamb	180 calories/3 oz.	Fatty lamb is significantly higher in calories.
Lean pork	225 calories/3 oz.	A good source of zinc, and one of the richest sources of thiamine (vitamin B_1). One of the best meat sources of vitamin B_{12}, too. Be judicious, though, and be sure it's lean.
Veal	185 calories/3 oz.	Generally lower in calories than sirloin. However, veal contains more cholesterol and more sodium than red meat. Be judicious.

How to Make These Foods Work for You

Now, just what do you do with all these fabulous foods—and intriguing insights? You gradually add a few well-chosen extras to your diet, using the Palm Beach Diet meal plans as your starting point. Your weight-maintenance diet will draw heavily on the foods listed here.

You want to maintain your goal weight, right? You can do so, given a few simple calculations. The first is to determine the number of calories which will halt weight loss, but prevent weight gain. In other words, you want to determine how much you can eat without jeopardizing your newly won shape!

You can do so easily. Most women fifty or more will find they can maintain their goal on 1300–1500 calories a day. Most mature men can have about 1600–1800 calories a day without gaining weight.

The Palm Beach Diet weighs in at roughly 1000–1200 calories a day. That means that women now can add about 300 calories per day and maintain their weight. Men can now enjoy about 500 more calories per day. Remember those numbers.

Monday of the Palm Beach Diet Core Week

MAINTENANCE ADDITIONS FOR WOMEN	MEALS	MAINTENANCE ADDITIONS FOR MEN
(1300–1500 calories/day total) Increase oatmeal to ⅔ cup and skim milk to ½ cup	**BREAKFAST** *Oatmeal (⅓ cup) topped with 1 tablespoon almonds and 1 tablespoon chopped dates* *¼ cup skim milk* *Coffee or tea, with skim milk and/or sugar substitute, if desired*	(1600–1800 calories/day total) Increase oatmeal to ⅔ cup and skim milk to ½ cup
	MID-MORNING SNACK *1 piece of fresh fruit—your choice* *Multivitamin/mineral supplement*	

	LUNCH *Palm Beach Salad in a whole-wheat pita pocket* *1 oz. Cheese* *Coffee or tea, with skim milk and/or sugar substitute, if desired*	Increase to 2 oz. cheese
Increase fish portion to 4 oz. Increase fettuccine portion to 3 oz. Add dinner roll with pat margarine	**DINNER** *Grouper Baked with Artichoke Hearts* *Spinach Fettuccine with Garlic* *1 cup broccoli* *2 pear halves (in ¼ cup orange juice, ground ginger)* *Coffee or tea, with skim milk and/or sugar substitute, if desired* *Remember your 6 glasses of water and your calcium supplement.*	Increase fish portion to 4 oz. Increase fettucine portion to 4 oz. Add dinner roll with pat margarine

Monday of the Palm Beach Diet Easy Week

MAINTENANCE ADDITIONS FOR WOMEN	MEALS	MAINTENANCE ADDITIONS FOR MEN
(1300–1500 calories/day total)	**BREAKFAST** *½ cup grapefruit juice* *An 8 oz. tub of plain, coffee, lemon or vanilla low-fat yogurt* *1 slice whole wheat toast* *1 teaspoon margarine* *Coffee or tea, with skim milk and/or sugar substitute, if desired*	(1600–1800 calories/day total)
Add 1 oz. package nuts and raisins	**MID-MORNING SNACK** *1 piece of fresh fruit—your choice* *Multiviamin/mineral supplement*	Add 2 oz. package nuts and raisins

	LUNCH	
Add a mid-afternoon snack of a banana or an apple	*Cup of vegetable soup* *Hard roll filled with 1 oz. Cheddar cheese, sliced tomato, lettuce and 1 teaspoon diet mayonnaise* *Coffee or tea, with skim milk and/or sugar substitute, if desired*	Add a mid-afternoon snack of a banana or an apple
	DINNER	
Increase fish portion to 6 oz. Add a granola bar for dessert	*3 oz. broiled white fish* *½ cup peas* *1 cup spinach, steamed* *1 tomato, sliced* *Whole wheat roll* *1 teaspoon butter or margarine* *Coffee or tea, with skim milk and/or sugar substitute, if desired.* *Remember your 6 glasses of water and your calcium supplement.*	Increase fish portion to 6 oz. Add a small side salad with low-calorie dressing Add a granola bar for dessert

Monday of the Palm Beach Diet "The Breakers" Week

MAINTENANCE ADDITIONS FOR WOMEN	MEALS	MAINTENANCE ADDITIONS FOR MEN
(1300–1500 calories/day total)	**BREAKFAST** *½ cup orange juice* *1 slice grilled bacon* *1 grilled tomato* *1 slice whole wheat toast* *1 teaspoon whipped sweet butter* *Tea or coffee with sugar substitute, if desired*	(1600–1800 calories/day total) Increase to ¾ cup orange juice Increase to 2 slices toast Increase to 2 teaspoons butter Add 2 teaspoons jam or marmalade
	MID-MORNING SNACK *½ cup fresh raspberries* *¾ cup skim milk* (*Multivitamin/mineral supplement per the Palm Beach Diet*)	

	LUNCH	
Add ⅓ cup cooked brown rice Add ½ cup sorbet or sherbet	*½ pink grapefruit* *6 medium shrimp, peeled and cooked, served on 2 slices of cucumber, 2 slices of tomato and leaves of Boston lettuce*	Add ⅓ cup cooked brown rice Increase to 4 slices melba toast
	Dressing: 1 teaspoon salad oil, 1 teaspoon red wine vinegar *2 slices melba toast* *¾ cup skim milk* *Coffee or iced tea with sugar substitute, if desired*	Add ½ cup sorbet or sherbet

(*continued*)

Monday of the Palm Beach Diet "The Breakers" Week

MAINTENANCE ADDITIONS FOR WOMEN	MEALS	MAINTENANCE ADDITIONS FOR MEN
	DINNER	
Increase veal chop to 4 oz.	*¾ cup consomme with 6 asparagus spears*	Increase veal chop to 4 oz.
	Broiled veal chop	
Increase to ¾ cup broccoli	*1 medium boiled potato*	Increase to ¾ cup broccoli
	1 medium grilled tomato	
Increase to ½ cup wine	*¼ cup broccoli*	Increase to ½ cup wine
Increase to 1 whole pear	*¼ cup white wine diluted with seltzer water*	Increase to 1 whole pear
Add a dinner roll	*½ pear*	Add a dinner roll
	10 grapes	
	Coffee or tea with sugar substitute, if desired	
	(6 glasses of water and calcium supplement per the Palm Beach Diet)	

Translating numbers into food isn't difficult. Let's take several days from the Palm Beach Diet and tack on 300 calories (for women) and 500 calories (for men). This will give you a feel for how to bump up calorie count without also bumping up your dress or trousers size! Note that in some cases, portion sizes have been increased to provide you with additional and healthy calories. In other instances, foods have been added.

Your Weight Maintenance Rules of Thumb

In the three sample days, we've added calories back to your diet—but intelligently. The increased portion sizes and additional foods suggested not only maintain your goal weight, they also maintain the biochemical balances important to you now, at fifty or more. They provide additional fiber, a little more protein and, in many cases, the sorts of complex carbohydrate foods which help to fill you up, so you don't feel hungry.

Perhaps the most important addition to your diet, now that you have calorie leeway, is fiber. The addition of such foods as rolls and bread, pasta, granola bars, nuts and fruit boost your fiber intake.

Additional protein is added primarily for satisfaction, generally at the evening meal. The rule of thumb: While dieting, you were allowed a 3- to 4-ounce portion of either fish, poultry or meat at dinner. As you continue to watch your weight, now that you've achieved your goal weight, you can increase your evening fish, poultry or meat serving to 3 to 6 ounces.

As you add calories back into your diet, too, remember to keep those two potential health nemeses in check: sodium and cholesterol. In the next chapter, you'll find listings of foods which contain significant levels of either sodium or cholesterol. Avoid these foods, especially in combination. The same caution should be extended to high-sugar, low-nutrient desserts. *Make them only an occasional treat.*

How to Order the Ideal Restaurant Meal

Eating out poses a problem to the dieter and the goal weight "maintainer" alike. Portion sizes, for example, are often scandalously large. There's the problem, too, of not knowing what you're getting: You may order a fish entree, for example, and find it comes sauced in cream and butter and ringed in creamed potato. Even the "honor roll" foods introduced in this chapter can become belt-loosening liabilities if the chef stresses quantity over quality or douses everything with butter.

I've noticed a trend here in Palm Beach which can help save you from the restaurant/calorie onslaught. This same approach to ordering a slimming yet satisfying meal in a restaurant is used wherever people dine out frequently and elegantly—as in Paris, New York and Los Angeles. The meal I'm about to describe, in fact, is a sort of international diet staple—appealing, satisfying and available at any good restaurant.

The meal starts with an optional glass of white wine, or mineral water with a twist of lime. The hors d'oeuvre is clear soup, such as consommé, or a piece of melon. The entree: broiled or lemon-baked fish, with vegetable and salad. Dessert, if desired, is sherbet or sorbet, or gingered fruit, accompanied by coffee or tea. If you choose not to have dessert, you may have a potato or rice with the entree instead. Watch sauces and dressings, remember. Top the potato with a squeeze of lemon juice, or a shake of Worcestershire sauce, not butter or sour cream. Keep the salad dressing simple: vinegar and oil, if possible. Typical "creamy Italian" house dressings are calorie-high. Avoid them. Ignore the bread basket, too!

For additional guidelines on restaurant dining, I couldn't turn to a better source than the American Heart Association's hints on eating out (© American Heart Association. Reproduced with permission):

IN THE MORNING: Breakfast need not be dull. Fish, chicken or lean meat provide a welcome change of pace. The variety of hot and cold cereals available is almost endless. Request low-fat milk instead of cream to use in coffee and cereal. Instead of an egg every day, limit eggs to two to three times a week. (Cut calories by asking for a poached or soft-cooked egg, thus avoiding the fat used in frying and scrambling.) Skip the Danishes and doughnuts in favor of English, corn or bran muffins or slices of whole wheat, rye or raisin bread toasted without butter. Request firmly that bread *not* be buttered, and ask that margarine be served at the table instead. Try a sprinkling of cinnamon *in place* of margarine. Fruit or juice of any variety is a delightful introduction or conclusion to the first meal of the day.

AT NOONTIME: For lunch, try a light meal such as a sandwich or salad. Try turkey, chicken, fish, large fruit or vegetable salads. For sandwiches, order lean meat, chicken, turkey or peanut butter. Avoid cold cuts. If you must choose between a grilled hamburger, hot dog or grilled cheese, select the hamburger.

Most salad dressings are high in calories. If oil and vinegar are available, mix your own using more vinegar than oil.

IN THE EVENING: Study the menu thoughtfully before ordering. Select food for quality, not quantity. An appetizer of melon, fish, tomato juice or a fresh vegetable platter is a wise choice. Ignore the liver paté, egg dishes and items prepared in cream sauces.

Thin broths and consommés are the best bets in the soup category; most other soups are made with a base of fatty meat stock or have a cream sauce base. For the entree, broiled, baked or roasted meat, fish, shellfish or poultry should take precedence over fried, grilled or sautéed versions of the same. When available, select the smaller portion. Limit your selection of shrimp and organ meats, which are high in cholesterol, to an occasional event. Duck and goose are taboo since they are too fatty. If fried or breaded foods are unavoidable, remove the outer crust and eat only the inside.

On request, chefs are usually willing to serve entrees without fatty sauces or gravies. It is a good idea to order your meat broiled specifically without butter, too.

You should not expect the chef to trim off every bit of visible fat, but you can do it yourself easily enough. If chicken or turkey is served intact, remove the skin before eating. Most of the fat in fowl is under the skin. As a general rule, dishes prepared in wine are acceptable. Those prepared in thick sauces and gravies, such as stews, are poor choices.

Vegetables pose little problem unless they are swimming in butter. Instruct the server accordingly. Go ahead and enjoy a baked potato, but skip the sour cream. For a new taste, try a dash of Worcestershire sauce or sprinkle a tablespoon of grated Parmesan cheese on the potato.

Ask that bread or rolls be served *with* the meal, not before. This not only prevents your filling up on bread, but cuts down on your use of butter or margarine. Remember, margarine, like butter, also adds calories.

The best choices for dessert are fruit, fruit ice, sherbet, gelatin and angel-food cake without icing. Forget whipped cream, whipped toppings and custard sauces.

An exotic finish to a gourmet meal is espresso or

demitasse coffee, black with a twist of lemon. Some may prefer to forego dessert in favor of brandy or a cordial, or even add a splash of anisette to demitasse.

Now you can see what I meant when I promised that you would not only learn how to lose weight, but learn how to keep weight off. You're fast becoming a discriminating—and slim—dieter, don't you agree? So let's not stop now. The next chapter is brimming with more tips and techniques.

CHAPTER 13

More New-Age Survival Tactics

You've mastered the restaurant meal. You know and enjoy the foods that maintain weight loss and support health. If you put this information into practice, you can remain in fine shape for years to come. I suggest that you refer to the last chapter from time to time, as you continue to refine your food choices and strengthen your commitment to healthy eating.

You may want to keep this chapter nearby, too, as a handy reference. Just as the last chapter identified your diet allies, this chapter names your enemies—foods which contain significant sodium or cholesterol, for example, and food additives which have not been "cleared" by adequate testing. You'll also learn your way around sometimes-deceptive food labeling, and dip into the psychology of food buying. Sometimes our brave new world can seem more daft than daring—especially to people who are fifty or more, and remember when the boast of "natural goodness" was more than an advertising slogan!

Staking Out Hidden Salt and Cholesterol

It's called "hidden" salt for a reason. It waits in ambush in foods. You may not realize that you're consuming salt at all.

We can hope that the Federal Food and Drug Administration will soon require that sodium content be listed on food labeling. This would be a big help to you—but only if you are in the habit of reading the nutritional information on food packaging. If you don't, you won't discover that, for example, a serving of canned soup can contain one-quarter of a day's healthy sodium allotment! Or that tuna packed in oil may contain 1.1 g. of sodium—again about one-quarter of a day's healthy sodium allotment. *Or* that corn flakes contain more salt ounce for ounce than cocktail peanuts! Then, too, fresh foods and some packaged foods aren't required to carry nutrient labeling, so it pays to know roughly which foods are sodium-low and which are very high in sodium.

Cholesterol is another bushwhacker. You are probably aware that eggs are high in cholesterol, but did you realize that chicken generally is higher in cholesterol than fish? That dark-meat chicken is higher in cholesterol than white-meat chicken? And that the cholesterol content of poultry can be lowered significantly by removing the skin, which contains the lion's share of cholesterol?

There's a move on today to get cholesterol content of foods on food labels. Currently, this information doesn't have to be included on ingredient labeling: When a food label does indicate cholesterol content, the manufacturer has provided the information voluntarily. And of course, produce, meats, poultry and fish rarely carry any form of nutrient labeling.

That's unhelpful to you, the consumer, of course. You have no alternative but to learn and remember those foods which are high in sodium or cholesterol. Here, then, is a helpful (although not all-inclusive) rundown of foods which contain relatively high amounts of sodium or cholesterol. Most of these foods shouldn't be eaten regularly, especially not along with others on the list. To do so oversteps the bounds of prudent sodium or cholesterol intake.

HIGH-CHOLESTEROL FOODS

The American Heart Association has recommended that Americans get less than 300 mg. of cholesterol per day.

Beef liver, 3 oz.	373 mg.
One egg	240 mg.
Squid, 3 oz.	153 mg.
Shrimp, 3 oz.	132 mg.
Chicken (dark meat, 3 oz.)	94 mg.
Veal, 3 oz.	83 mg.
Oily fish, 3 oz.	69 mg.
Ice cream, 1 cup	56 mg.
Clams (6 large)	55 mg.
Lean fish, 3 oz.	51 mg.
Lean beef, 3 oz.	51 mg.
Whole milk, 1 cup	34 mg.
Cheddar cheese, 1 oz.	28 mg.
Parmesan cheese, 1 oz.	27 mg.
American cheese, 1 oz.	26 mg.
Low-fat yogurt, 1 cup	17 mg.
Butter, 1 tablespoon	12 mg.

Sodium, incidentally, goes by many aliases. These salt pseudonyms include: sodium bicarbonate, brine, caseinate, citrate, chloride, phosphate, propionate and nitrate. Any food ingredient which contains the word "sodium" *is* also salt: Sodium benzoate and monosodium glutamate are examples. If any of these items ranks high on an ingredient label, that food may be quite salty.

HIGH-SALT FOODS

Asparagus	Milk chocolate
Bacon	Mustard
Baking powder	Oatmeal (flavored, in packets)
Beets (canned)	Olives
Bouillon	Oysters (frozen)
Broth	Peas (canned)
Butter (salted)	Pickles
Calf's liver	Many pie fillings
Caviar	Pizza
Carrots (canned)	Potato chips
Catsup	Pretzels
Many cereals	Many ready-to-eat dinners
Cheese (except reduced salt	Relish
Chili sauce	Salmon (canned, pink)
Corn (canned)	Salted crackers
Corned beef (canned)	Salted popcorn
Corn chips	Salted nuts
Frozen dinners	Sardines (canned)
Garlic salt	Sauerkraut
Gravy mixes	Sausage
Green beans (canned)	Self-rising flour
Ham	Many canned soups
Hot dogs	Soy sauce
Lima beans	Tomatoes (canned)
Lobster	Tomato juice (canned)
Luncheon meats	Tuna (canned in oil)
Margarine (salted)	Worcestershire sauce
Milk	

(Sugar, too, goes by aliases, including this long list of substances: brown sugar, corn syrup, dextrose, galactose, glucose, honey, invert sugar, lactose, maltose, maple syrup, molasses, raw sugar, sucrose and turbinado. Excessive sugar has no business in your diet, either: If any of these names appears high on the ingredient labeling of a food you're considering buying, consider putting it back on the shelf!)

Tapping into the Psychology of Food Buying

Another way you can wind up with unintended items in your kitchen cupboard: Buying food items you don't really want or need. "It looked so good," you tell yourself later. Meanwhile, that impulse buy—very likely loaded either with fat or sugar—has padded your hips, distended your stomach and overstretched your food budget.

Americans spend over $3 billion a year on food and drink. We could cut that bill by a whopping 70 percent by shopping smartly. Impulse buying is one area of food budget indiscretion. And you can bet that grocery stores and supermarkets take advantage of the psychology of food buying.

On your next visit to the market, notice the way in which products are distributed throughout the store. Staples are generally located in different aisles; meats may be sold at one end of the store, and produce at the other. In order to gather your staples, in other words, you must wheel past shelves and displays of enticing yet dispensable goodies.

Another consumer trap: High-profit items often are placed near companion staples, while less expensive alternatives are located elsewhere. Example: Expensive salad dressings may be located in a display over the lettuce—while cheaper dressings, oils and vinegars are five aisles away.

Products placed at the end of aisles, and close to the cash register, are especially visible. It's easy to assume that these prominently displayed items are sale items. Don't assume! And remember: You're a sitting duck, too, for last-minute impulse purchases at the cash register. The racks of candies there may tempt you—but resist the urge. Beat both the system and weight gain.

As you're shopping, remember to compare unit prices of items. Bigger isn't necessarily cheaper! While you can save on most groceries and household staples by choosing the large "economy" or "family" size over convenience sizes, there are many exceptions to this rule. Items that sometimes are *more* expensive, by unit, in larger sizes include powdered bleaches and detergents, dishwashing liquids, tomato sauce, salad oils, tuna, all-purpose flour, instant tea with lemon and sugar, and coffee. What's up? Perhaps it has to do with the slower turnover rate of outsized products. At any rate, unit pricing is an easy way to compare brands and package sizes for value.

Feeding Food Paranoia: "All Natural" vs. "Artificial"

Nothing sells like "natural." The word invites consumer confidence, according to one national survey. But does "natural" really mean that a product so labeled is fresh, wholesome, and free of additives? Is it somehow better than a similar item that doesn't wave the word "natural" like a banner on its label?

Not necessarily. The term "natural flavor," for example, may be used on foods as long as natural flavors *predominate.* The boast "natural flavors" does *not* guarantee that artificial flavors aren't also included in the product.

Some foods also use the term "natural" rather loosely. The Food, Drug and Cosmetic Act of 1938 exempts certain common foods from ingredient labeling. Such foods as cheeses, cheese products, egg products, mayonnaise, ice cream and bakery goods needn't carry ingredient labeling *if* they conform to what's termed a "Standard of Identity"—an established "recipe" for a particular kind of food. The standard for mayonnaise, for example, mandates that the product contain 65 percent, by weight, of vegetable oil, plus vinegar or lemon juice, and egg yolk. So far, that makes mayonnaise a "natural" product, all right. Here's the catch, however—as long as the standard is met, manufacturers can then add other ingredients to the product, and still boast of naturalness—even if the additional ingredients are stabilizers or preservatives, for example. Hence, "all natural" ice cream may contain stabilizers and additives.

The word "fortified" may be misleading, too. Fortification of breads, and cereals in some cases, *is* a good idea. Often, however, the boast of fortification is a ruse to make junk foods appear nutritious. A "fortified" drink, for example, may claim to have more vitamin C than orange juice or more iron than milk. (Milk is not a good iron source anyway, so the comparison is moot.) Meanwhile, the fortified product also may contain a lot of sugar, artificial flavoring, artificial coloring and preservatives.

Sometimes, too, it pays to beware the popular banner blazed across a jar: "No Artificial Preservatives." It could mean the product costs considerably more than a conventional version of the same food—and yet contains exactly the same components. How is that possible? Many *natural* food substances are good preservatives—sugar and salt are food life-extenders, for example. A jar of jam or a bottle of juice which claims to have "no artificial preservatives" may contain the same natural sugar or salt preservative as the jam or juice next to it on the shelf. And cost a lot more.

A little perspective on the "natural" vs. "artificial" skirmish may be in order. Sure, the fervor for natural foods is a healthy trend; most foods are more nutritious the more closely they resemble their original form. It's not the "natural" that bestows health benefits in many cases, however; it's the *freshness* and the *lack of processing or refining.* Preserved foods also happen to be the ones most likely to have undergone a refining process which compromises nutrients. Rather than hunt for the word "natural"—and pay more, I'd prefer to see you gravitate toward fresh foods and those which haven't been processed—old-fashioned oatmeal, for example, rather than flavored oatmeal. (The latter generally contains added salt, and costs more than the old-fashioned form.) So remember: "fresh" and "unrefined" are more relevant buzz words than "natural."

Additives—What About Them?

Artificial additives, meanwhile, are a continuing source of controversy. Indeed, there have been food additive scares, and subsequent quick removal of suspect foods from the marketplace. And it's true that some additives haven't yet been tested thoroughly: We can't state with authority that they're safe or unsafe. Still, most of the additives in foods today are safe: A few exceptions to the rule have created a backlash against all food additives.

The truth is that the health-risks associated with unhygienic or ill-preserved foods are higher than risks associated with most food additives. Once more, many of the artificial food additives in use today are no more risky than the *natural* toxins in natural foods. For example, cabbage, broccoli and shallots contain antithyroid, gout-promoting compounds. Shrimp contains arsenic. Potato contains arsenic and nitrate—nitrate is the preservative the public has been told to avoid in hot dogs and bacon!

I'm not suggesting that you ignore the fresh foods cited here. My point is that almost every food contains toxins in minute, and generally harmless, amounts. You would have to consume extraordinary amounts of foods that contain traces of toxins over years or decades of time before a toxic effect would show up. Even then, in most cases, you wouldn't be threatened with toxicity. According to Martha E. Rhodes, head of the Food Laboratory, Division of Chemistry of Florida's Department of Agriculture and Consumer Services: "The toxicities of chemicals in our diet do not supplement each other and are not additive, and often the toxic effects of one chemical offsets the effects of another: for example, iodine (in seafood and table salt) offsets the effects of goitrogens (gout-promoting substances) found in some vegetables."

As a consumer, you need remember two things, then, to safeguard against toxicity from foods. The first: *Your best defense against consuming significant levels of any toxic substance, be it "artificial" or "natural," is to eat a varied diet.* Don't overdo on any one food or any one food group. For example, it's prudent to limit yourself to one saccharin-sweetened can of diet soda a day, and to limit such items as cold cuts, ham, hot dogs and bacon—all of which contain nitrates—to once or twice a week. Your second defense: Avoiding food substances that either have not been tested adequately, or remain controversial.

The chart that follows shows you how. It was compiled by the Center for Science in the Public Interest, a nonprofit organization based in Washington, D.C., which seeks to protect consumers' interest in matters of public food and health policy. The chart names common food additives and suggests which are safe, which should be avoided (because they are unsafe in the amounts consumed or have been very poorly tested), and which food additives should be used with caution (the additive may be unsafe, is poorly tested or is used in foods we tend to eat too much of).

FOOD ADDITIVES

The common food additives below are described, and assigned either a * to indicate safety, an **X** to indicate that a particular additive should be avoided, or a **?** to indicate caution should be used—don't use that particular substance in large quantities.

*	ALGINATE, PROPYLENE GLYCOL ALGINATE Thickening agents; foam stabilizer *Ice cream, cheese, candy, yogurt*	Alginate, an apparently safe derivative of seaweed (kelp), maintains the desired texture in dairy products, canned frosting, and other factory-made foods. Propylene glycol alginate, a chemically modified algin, thickens acidic foods (soda pop, salad dressing) and stabilizes the foam in beer.
*	ALPHA TOCOPHEROL (Vitamin E) Antioxidant, nutrient *Vegetable oil*	Vitamin E is abundant in whole wheat, rice germ, and vegetable oils. It is destroyed by the refining and bleaching of flour. Vitamin E prevents oils from going rancid.

ARTIFICIAL COLORINGS

Most artificial colorings are synthetic chemicals that do not occur in nature. Though some are safer than others, colorings are not listed by name on labels. Because colorings are used almost solely in foods of low nutritional value (candy, soda pop, gelatin desserts, etc.), you should simply avoid all artificially colored foods. In addition to problems mentioned below, there is evidence that colorings may cause hyperactivity in some sensitive children. The use of coloring usually indicates that fruit or other natural ingredient has not been used.

X	BLUE No. 1 Artificial coloring *Beverages, candy, baked goods*	Inadequately tested; suggestions of a small cancer risk. Avoid.
X	BLUE No. 2 Artificial coloring *Pet food, beverages, candy*	The largest, most recent study suggested but did not prove that this dye caused brain tumors in male mice. The FDA concluded that there is "reasonable certainty of no harm."

(*continued*)

X	CITRUS RED No. 2 Artificial coloring *Skin of some Florida oranges only*	Studies indicate that this additive causes cancer. The dye does not seep through the orange skin into the pulp.
X	GREEN No. 3 Artificial coloring *Candy, beverages*	A 1981 industry-sponsored study gave hints of bladder cancer, but FDA re-analyzed the data using other statistical tests and concluded that the dye was safe. Fortunately, this possibly carcinogenic dye is rarely used.
X	RED No. 3 Artificial coloring *Cherries in fruit cocktail, candy, baked goods*	The evidence that this dye causes thyroid tumors in rats is "convincing," according to a 1983 review committee report requested by FDA. There are also suggestions that it may affect the brain and behavior. Avoid.
?	RED No. 40 Artificial coloring *Soda pop, candy, gelatin desserts, pastry, pet food, sausage*	The most widely used food dye. While this is one of the most tested food dyes, the key mouse tests were flawed and inconclusive. An FDA review committee acknowledged problems, but said evidence of harm was not "consistent" or "substantial." Like other dyes, Red No. 40 is used mainly in junk foods.
?	YELLOW No. 5 Artificial coloring *Gelatin dessert, candy, pet food, baked goods*	The second most widely used coloring causes allergic reactions, primarily in aspirin-sensitive persons. This dye is the only one that must be labeled by name on food labels.
?	YELLOW No. 6 Artificial coloring *Beverages, sausage, baked goods, candy, gelatin*	Appears safe, but can cause occasional allergic reactions; used almost exclusively in junk foods.

?	ARTIFICIAL FLAVORING Flavoring *Soda pop, candy, breakfast cereals, gelatin desserts; many others*	Hundreds of chemicals are used to mimic natural flavors; many may be used in a single flavoring, such as for cherry soda pop. Most flavoring chemicals also occur in nature and are probably safe, but they may cause hyperactivity in some sensitive children. Artificial flavorings are used almost exclusively in junk foods; their use indicates that the real thing (usually fruit) has been left out.
*	ASCORBIC ACID (Vitamin C), ERYTHORBIC ACID Antioxidant, nutrient, color stabilizer *Oily foods, cereals, soft drinks, cured meats*	ASCORBIC ACID helps maintain the red color of cured meat and prevents the formation of nitrosamines (see *sodium nitrite*). It helps prevent loss of color and flavor by reacting with unwanted oxygen. It is used as a nutrient additive in drinks and breakfast cereals. SODIUM ASCORBATE is a more soluble form of ascorbic acid. ERYTHORBIC ACID (sodium erythorbate) serves the same functions as ascorbic acid, but has no value as a vitamin.
?	ASPARTAME Artificial sweetener *Drink mixes, gelatin desserts, other foods*	ASPARTAME, made up of two amino acids, was thought to be the perfect artificial sweetener, but questions have arisen about the quality of the cancer tests and persons have reported severe adverse behavioral effects after drinking diet soda. If you use aspartame, be careful! People with PKU need to avoid it, also.
*	BETA CAROTENE Coloring; nutrient *Margarine, shortening, nondairy whiteners, butter*	Used as an artificial coloring and a nutrient supplement. The body converts it to vitamin A, which is part of the light-detection mechanism of the eye.

(*continued*)

X	BROMINATED VEGETABLE OIL (BVO) Emulsifier, clouding agent *Soft drinks*	BVO keeps flavor oils in suspension and gives a cloudy appearance to citrus-flavored soft drinks. The residues of BVO found in body fat are cause for concern. BVO should be banned; safer substitutes are available.
X	BUTYLATED HYDROXYANISOLE (BHA) Antioxidant *Cereals, chewing gum, potato chips, vegetable oil*	BHA retards rancidity in fats, oils, and oil-containing foods. While most studies indicate it is safe, a 1982 Japanese study demonstrated that it caused cancer in rats. This synthetic chemical can often be replaced by safer chemicals.
X	BUTYLATED HYDROXYTOLUENE (BHT) Antioxidant *Cereals, chewing gum, potato chips, oils, etc.*	BHT retards rancidity in oils. It either increased or decreased the risk of cancer in various animal studies. Residues of BHT occur in human fat. BHT is unnecessary or is easily replaced by safe substitutes. Avoid it when possible.
X	CAFFEINE Stimulant *Coffee, tea, cocoa* (*natural*); *soft drinks* (*additive*)	Caffeine may cause miscarriages or birth defects and should be avoided by pregnant women. It also keeps many people from sleeping. New evidence indicates that caffeine may cause fibrocystic breast disease in some women.
*	CALCIUM (or SODIUM) PROPIONATE Preservative *Bread, rolls, pies, cakes*	CALCIUM PROPIONATE prevents mold growth on bread and rolls. The calcium is a beneficial mineral; the propionate is safe. SODIUM PROPIONATE is used in pies and cakes, because calcium alters the action of chemical leavening agents.
*	CALCIUM (or SODIUM) STEAROYL LACTYLATE Dough conditioner,	These additives strengthen bread dough so it can be used in bread-making machinery and lead to more uniform grain and greater volume. They act as whip-

	whipping agent *Bread dough, cake fillings, artificial whipped cream, processed egg whites*	ping agents in dried, liquid, or frozen egg whites and artificial whipped cream. SODIUM STEAROYL FUMARATE serves the same function.
?	CARRAGEENAN Thickening and stabilizing agent *Ice cream, jelly, chocolate milk, infant formula*	Carrageenan is obtained from seaweed. Large amounts of carrageenan have harmed test animals' colons; the small amounts in food are probably safe. Needs better tests.
*	CASEIN, SODIUM CASEINATE Thickening and whitening agent *Ice cream, ice milk, sherbet, coffee creamers*	Casein, the principal protein in milk, is a nutritious protein containing adequate amounts of all the essential amino acids.
*	CITRIC ACID, SODIUM CITRATE Acid, flavoring, chelating agent *Ice creams, sherbet, fruit drink, candy, carbonated beverages, instant potatoes*	CITRIC ACID is versatile, widely used, cheap, and safe. It is an important metabolite in virtually all living organisms; especially abundant in citrus fruits and berries. It is used as a strong acid, a tart flavoring, and an antioxidant. SODIUM CITRATE, also safe, is a buffer that controls the acidity of gelatin desserts, jam, ice cream, candy, and other foods.
?	CORN SYRUP Sweetener, thickener *Candy, toppings, syrups, snack foods, imitation dairy foods*	Corn syrup is a sweet, thick liquid made by treating cornstarch with acids or enzymes. It may be dried and used as CORN SYRUP SOLIDS in coffee whiteners, and other dry products. Corn syrup contains no nutritional value other than calories, promotes tooth decay, and is used mainly in low-nutrition foods.

(*continued*)

?	DEXTROSE (GLUCOSE, CORN SUGAR) Sweetener, coloring agent *Bread, caramel, soda pop, cookies, many other foods*	Dextrose is an important chemical in every living organism. A sugar, it is a source of sweetness in fruits and honey. Added to foods as a sweetener, it represents empty calories, and contributes to tooth decay. Dextrose turns brown when heated and contributes to the color of bread crust and toast.
*	EDTA Chelating agent *Salad dressing, margarine, sandwich spreads, mayonnaise, processed fruits and vegetables, canned shellfish, soft drinks*	Modern food manufacturing technology, which involves metal rollers, blenders, and containers, results in trace amounts of metal contamination in food. EDTA (ethylenediamine tetraacetic acid) traps metal impurities, which would otherwise promote rancidity and the breakdown of artificial colors.
*	FERROUS GLUCONATE Coloring, nutrient *Black olives*	Used by the olive industry to generate a uniform jet-black color and in pills as a source of iron. Safe.
*	FUMARIC ACID Tartness agent *Powdered drinks, pudding, pie fillings, gelatin desserts*	A solid at room temperature, inexpensive, highly acidic, it is the ideal source of tartness and acidity in dry food products. However, it dissolves slowly in cold water, a drawback cured by adding DIOCTYL SODIUM SULFOSUCCINATE (DSS), a poorly tested, detergent-like additive.
*	GELATIN Thickening and gelling agent *Powdered dessert mix, yogurt, ice cream, cheese spreads, beverages*	Gelatin is a protein obtained from animal bones, hoofs, and other parts. It has little nutritional value, because it contains little or none of several essential amino acids.
*	GLYCERIN (GLYCEROL) Maintains water	Glycerin forms the backbone of fat and oil molecules and is quite safe. The body uses it as a source of energy or as a

	content *Marshmallow, candy, fudge, baked goods*	starting material in making more complex molecules.
*	GUMS: Guar, Locust Bean, Arabic, Furcelleran, Ghatti, Karaya, Tragacanth Thickening agents, stabilizers *Beverages, ice cream, frozen pudding, salad dressing, dough, cottage cheese, candy, drink mixes*	Gums derive from natural sources (bushes, trees, or seaweed) and are poorly tested. They are used to thicken foods, prevent sugar crystals from forming in candy, stabilize beer foam (arabic), form a gel in pudding (furcelleran), encapsulate flavor oils in powdered drink mixes, or keep oil and water mixed together in salad dressings. Tragacanth, sometimes used in McDonald's "Big Macs" and many other foods, has caused occasional severe allergic reactions.
?	HEPTYL PARABEN Preservative *Beer, non-carbonated soft drinks*	Heptyl paraben—short for the heptyl ester of parahydroxybenzoic acid—is a preservative. Studies suggest this chemical is safe, but it, like other additives in alcoholic beverages, has never been tested in the presence of alcohol.
?	HYDROGENATED VEGETABLE OIL Source of oil or fat *Margarine, many processed foods*	Vegetable oil, usually a liquid, can be made into a semisolid by treating with hydrogen. Unfortunately, hydrogenation converts some of the polyunsaturated oil to saturated fat. We eat too much oil and fat of all kinds, whether natural or hydrogenated. High fat diets promote heart disease, obesity, and probably cancer.
*	HYDROLYZED VEGETABLE PROTEIN (HVP) Flavor enhancer *Instant soups, frankfurters, sauce mixes, beef stew*	HVP consists of vegetable (usually soybean) protein that has been chemically broken down to the amino acids of which it is composed. HVP is used to bring out the natural flavor of food (and, perhaps, to use less real food).

(*continued*)

?	INVERT SUGAR Sweetener *Candy, soft drinks, many other foods*	Invert sugar, a 50–50 mixture of two sugars, dextrose and fructose, is sweeter and more soluble than sucrose (table sugar). Invert sugar forms when sucrose is split in two by an enzyme or acid. It represents "empty calories," contributes to tooth decay, and should be avoided.
*	LACTIC ACID Acidity regulator *Spanish olives, cheese, frozen desserts, carbonated beverages*	This safe acid occurs in almost all living organisms. It inhibits spoilage in Spanish-type olives, balances the acidity in cheese-making, and adds tartness to frozen desserts, carbonated fruit-flavored drinks, and other foods.
*	LACTOSE Sweetener *Whipped topping mix, breakfast pastry*	Lactose, a carbohydrate found only in milk, is Nature's way of delivering calories to infant mammals. One-sixth as sweet as table sugar, it is added to food as a slightly sweet source of carbohydrate. Milk turns sour when bacteria convert lactose to lactic acid. Many non-Caucasians have trouble digesting lactose.
*	LECITHIN Emulsifier, antioxidant *Baked goods, margarine, chocolate, ice cream*	A common constituent of animal and plant tissues, it is a source of the nutrient choline. It keeps oil and water from separating out, retards rancidity, reduces spattering in a frying pan, and leads to fluffier cakes. Major sources are egg yolk and soybeans.
*	MANNITOL Sweetener, other uses *Chewing gum, low-calorie foods*	Not quite as sweet as sugar and poorly absorbed by the body, it contributes only half as many calories as sugar. Used as the "dust" on chewing gum, it prevents gum from absorbing moisture and becoming sticky. Safe.
*	MONO- and DIGLYCERIDES Emulsifier	Makes bread softer and prevents staling, improves the stability of margarine, makes caramels less sticky, and pre-

Baked goods, margarine, candy, peanut butter	vents the oil in peanut butter from separating out. Mono- and diglycerides are safe, though most foods they are used in are high in refined flour, sugar, or fat.
? MONOSODIUM GLUTAMATE (MSG) Flavor enhancer *Soup, seafood, poultry, cheese, sauces, stews; many others*	This amino acid brings out the flavor of protein-containing foods. Large amounts of MSG fed to infant mice destroyed nerve cells in the brain. Public pressure forced baby food companies to stop using MSG. MSG causes "Chinese Restaurant Syndrome" (burning sensation in the back of neck and forearms, tightness of the chest, headache) in some sensitive adults.
? PHOSPHORIC ACID; PHOSPHATES Acidulant, chelating agent, buffer, emulsifier, nutrient, discoloration inhibitor *Baked goods, cheese, powdered foods, cured meat, soda pop, breakfast cereals, dehydrated potatoes*	PHOSPHORIC ACID acidifies and flavors cola beverages. Phosphate salts are used in hundreds of processed foods for many purposes. CALCIUM and IRON PHOSPHATES act as mineral supplements. SODIUM ALUMINUM PHOSPHATE is a leavening agent. CALCIUM AND AMMONIUM PHOSPHATES serve as food for yeast in bread. SODIUM ACID PYROPHOSPHATE prevents discoloration in potatoes and sugar syrups. Phosphates are not toxic, but their widespread use has led to dietary imbalances that may be contributing to osteoporosis.
* POLYSORBATE 60 Emulsifier *Baked goods, frozen desserts, imitation dairy products*	POLYSORBATE 60 is short for polyoxyethylene—(20)—sorbitan monostearate. It and its close relatives, POLYSORBATE 65 and 80, work the same way as mono- and diglycerides, but smaller amounts are needed. They keep baked goods from going stale, keep dill oil dissolved in bottled dill pickles, help coffee whiteners dissolve in coffee, and prevent oil from separating out of artificial whipped cream.

(*continued*)

X	PROPYL GALLATE Antioxidant *Vegetable oil, meat products, potato sticks, chicken soup base, chewing gum*	Retards the spoilage of fats and oils and is often used with BHA and BHT, because of the synergistic effect these additives have. The best long-term feeding study (1981) was peppered with suggestions (but not proof) of cancer. Avoid.
X	QUININE Flavoring *Tonic water, quinine water, bitter lemon*	This drug can cure malaria and is used as a bitter flavoring in a few soft drinks. There is a slight chance that quinine may cause birth defects, so pregnant women should avoid quinine-containing beverages and drugs. Very poorly tested.
X	SACCHARIN Synthetic sweetener *"Diet" products*	Saccharin is 350 times sweeter than sugar. Studies have not shown that saccharin helps people lose weight. In 1977, the FDA proposed that saccharin be banned, because of repeated evidence that it causes cancer. It is gradually being replaced by aspartame (NutraSweet). Avoid.
X	SALT (SODIUM CHLORIDE) Flavoring *Most processed foods: soup, potato chips, crackers*	Salt is used liberally in many processed foods. Other additives contribute additional sodium. A diet high in sodium may cause high blood pressure, which increases the risk of heart attack and stroke. Everyone should eat less salt: avoid salty processed foods, use salt sparingly, enjoy other seasonings.
*	SODIUM BENZOATE *Fruit juice, carbonated drinks, pickles, preserves*	Manufacturers have used sodium benzoate for over 70 years to prevent the growth of microorganisms in acidic foods.

*	SODIUM CARBOXY-METHYLCELLULOSE (CMC) Thickening and stabilizing agent; prevents sugar from crystallizing *Ice cream, beer, pie fillings, icings, diet foods, candy*	CMC is made by reacting cellulose with a derivative of acetic acid. Studies indicate it is safe.
X	SODIUM NITRITE, SODIUM NITRATE Preservative, coloring, flavoring *Bacon, ham, frankfurters, luncheon meats, smoked fish, corned beef*	NITRITE can lead to the formation of small amounts of potent cancer-causing chemicals (nitrosamines), particularly in fried bacon. Nitrite is tolerated in foods because it can prevent the growth of bacteria that cause botulism poisoning. Nitrite also stabilizes the red color in cured meat and gives a characteristic flavor. Companies should find safer methods of preventing botulism. Meanwhile, *don't bring home the bacon.* SODIUM NITRATE is used in dry cured meat, because it slowly breaks down into nitrite.
*	SORBIC ACID, POTASSIUM SORBATE Prevents growth of mold and bacteria *Cheese, syrup, jelly, cake, wine, dry fruits*	SORBIC ACID occurs naturally in the berries of the mountain ash. SORBATE may be a safe replacement for sodium nitrite in bacon. If potassium sorbate is more widely used, it should be tested more fully.
*	SORBITAN MONOSTEARATE Emulsifier *Cakes, candy, frozen pudding, icing*	Like mono- and diglycerides and polysorbates, this additive keeps oil and water mixed together. In chocolate candy, it prevents the discoloration that normally occurs when the candy is warmed up and then cooled down.

(*continued*)

*	SORBITOL Sweetener, thickening agent, maintains moisture *Dietetic drinks and foods; candy, shredded coconut, chewing gum*	Sorbitol occurs naturally in fruits and berries and is a close relative of the sugars. It is half as sweet as sugar. It is used in non-cariogenic chewing gum because oral bacteria do not metabolize it well. Large amounts of sorbitol (2 oz. for adults) have a laxative effect, but otherwise it is safe. Diabetics use sorbitol, because it is absorbed slowly and does not cause blood sugar to increase rapidly.
*	STARCH, MODIFIED STARCH Thickening agent *Soup, gravy, baby foods*	Starch, the major component of flour, potatoes, and corn, is used as a thickening agent. However, it does not dissolve in cold water. Chemists have solved this problem by reacting starch with various chemicals. These modified starches are added to some foods to improve their consistency and keep the solids suspended. Starch and modified starches make foods look thicker and richer than they really are.
X	SUGAR (SUCROSE) Sweetener *Table sugar, sweetened foods*	Sucrose, ordinary table sugar, occurs naturally in fruit, sugar cane, and sugar beets. Americans consume about 100 pounds of refined sugar per year. Sugar makes up about one-sixth of the average diet, but contains no vitamins, minerals, or protein. Sugar and sweetened foods may taste good and supply energy, but most people eat too much of them. Unless you enjoy large dentist bills and a large waistline, you should eat much less sugar.
X	SULFUR DIOXIDE, SODIUM BISULFITE Preservative, bleach *Sliced fruit, wine, grape juice, dehydrated potatoes*	Sulfiting agents prevent discoloration (some restaurant salads, dried fruit) and bacterial growth (wine). They also destroy vitamin B_1 and can cause severe allergic reactions, especially in asthmatics. Avoid this food additive since it has been known to cause death.

* VANILLIN, ETHYL VANILLIN Substitute for vanilla *Ice cream, baked goods, beverages, chocolate, candy, gelatin desserts*	Vanilla flavoring is derived from a bean, but VANILLIN, the major flavor component of vanilla, is cheaper to produce in a factory. A derivative, ETHYL VANILLIN, comes closer to matching the taste of real vanilla. Both chemicals are safe.

Additives: The Good, the Bad, the So-So

The message of the Food Additives chart: Consumer be aware! Be aware not only of certain questionable food additives, but also of those which are safe, and *needn't* be avoided in a health-conscious diet. I don't want you paying higher prices for "health foods" which are not necessarily more healthy than conventional versions of the same item.

This is an important point to make among people who are fifty or more. America's older population is the biggest consumer of "health foods." Mature individuals, hoping to hedge against old age and illness, are vulnerable to overpricing and inflated health-food claims. They are likely to use "natural" foods, and such substances as dolomite, kelp, bone meal, dessicated beef liver, ginseng and herbal teas in lieu of medical care. That is not a good idea. In fact, some of these so-called "health foods" can be unhealthy. Ginseng can raise blood pressure; dessicated beef liver powder is sometimes contaminated with salmonella bacteria, which can produce gastroenteritis. Beef liver is also high in cholesterol. Kelp is high in sodium. Some herbal teas—notably sassafras and chamomile—can have undesirable side effects. I've already described the potential dangers of dolomite and bone meal elsewhere. Again: Consumer be aware!

Some At-Home Help

You've chosen foods that are as fresh as possible; you're judicious in your use of foods that are refined and processed. You're half-way home. Now, how you store and cook your healthy fare at home will determine its ultimate nutrient content. *Fact:* You can select the choicest produce, fish, poultry and meats and then weaken them nutritionally through haphazard storing and cooking methods at home. Since I *know* you want to derive all of the health benefits of the Palm Beach Diet, here are some tips on safeguarding the vitamin content of your foods. You don't have to fuss. In most cases, you just have to use common sense.

Storing and Cooking Fruits and Vegetables

The vitamins within fruits and vegetables are often severely compromised by long storage times and by overcooking. For these reasons, the Palm Beach Diet advocates the freshest fruits and vegetables possible, and recommends steaming or microwaving vegetables. Steaming and microwaving reduce or eliminate the leeching of vitamins which occurs with boiling, frying, baking and sautéeing.

Don't throw away the most nutritious portion of vegetables! Leave skin on salad vegetables when possible: The skin of a cucumber, for example, contains most of the nutrients. Don't discard the leaves of broccoli stalks—they're nutrient-rich. The outer and generally greener leaves of cabbage and lettuces have a higher vitamin content than do the paler inner leaves.

Spare the vitamin content of vegetables the following ways:

Vitamin A: A little-known fact is that cooking vegetables which contain vitamin A increases the availability of the vitamin A to the body. Cooking compromises vitamins B and C, however, so steer a middle course—cook until just tender.

Vitamin B: Wash fruit and vegetables quickly before eating or cooking, as the B vitamins and vitamin C are lost by the act of rinsing. Don't add a pinch of baking soda to cooking vegetables to brighten their color—a common practice: Alkaline substances such as baking soda destroy vitamin B_1 (thiamine). The B vitamins (and vitamin C as well) are easily lost by overcooking. Use as little water as possible when cooking vegetables and fruits. Again, steaming and microwaving are ideal cooking methods.

Vitamin C: Vitamin C is lost in vegetables and fruits which are skin-damaged. Time is a vitamin C antagonist, too: Buy fresh and store in a refrigerator. If you don't plan to use a vegetable for several days, either buy under-ripe or choose a frozen variety.

As soon as you cut into vegetables or fruits, they begin to lose vitamin C. Don't prepare salads in advance, for example, and let them sit for an hour or more while you prepare the remainder of the meal. Make a fresh salad at the *last* possible minute. When you cut into cantaloupe or honeydew melon and serve just a portion of it, wrap the other portion tightly in airtight wrap. Do the same for all vegetable and fruit leftovers such as partially used tomatoes, heads of lettuce, kiwi fruit slices, etc.

Canned fruits and vegetables preserve vitamin C, incidentally. Canning destroys the enzyme which destroys vitamin C—thus *sparing* vitamin C. Here's a reason, too, for chilling fresh fruits and vegetables as soon after picking as possible: This vitamin C-destroying enzyme is inactivated by cold temperatures.

Choosing and Using Bread

Bread defies the "fresh is best" rule. Day-old bread is as nutritious as fresh-baked.

Throughout these pages, I've pitched for "whole grain" and "whole wheat" breads; both guarantee the goodness of the entire grain—the outer bran layer, the central endosperm and the inner germ. By now you've learned that whole grain bread and whole wheat bread are more nutritious than white bread. You have to pick your way through the labels, though, to know what you're getting!

Don't be misled by either of the following attributions, for instance: The first: "fiber fortified." It may mean that a fiber called wood cellulose has been added to the bread; unlike the fiber in grains, vegetables and fruits, wood cellulose absorbs very little water. That, in turn, means that it doesn't bulk up during digestion, and doesn't offer the health benefits of vegetable fiber. Once more, the long-term effects of consuming wood pulp are unknown. You've probably been faced before with burnt toast—but never the prospect of splintered toast!

"Enriched" is another high-sounding attribution that makes bread appear especially good for you. Enriched bread has been stripped of nutrients during the refining process, however, and then refortified with B vitamins and iron. The bread may well be deficient in such minerals as zinc, chromium and magnesium—minerals left intact in whole grain bread and whole wheat bread.

Lesson: Look for bread which is whole grain or whole wheat, and states so clearly on the label.

An aside on pasta: It's common practice to store pasta in pretty glass containers and display them on a kitchen shelf or counter. This practice, however, destroys the vitamin B_2 (riboflavin) in pasta, as fluorescent light penetrates glass and destroys riboflavin. Store pasta instead in opaque jars, or leave your pasta in its cardboard boxes in the cupboard.

Choosing and Using Milk

The riboflavin in milk may be destroyed by leaving milk in glass containers under fluorescent light, or in sunlight. Choose opaque or cardboard containers *or* keep milk away from light altogether.

On the Palm Beach Diet, you're asked to use skim milk. Skim milk contains about half the calories of whole milk. Dried skim milk is also acceptable—and may help alleviate the gassy reaction to milk that some people experience.

For the record, milk which boasts of being "1 percent fat" or "2 percent fat" is not 99 or 98 percent freer of fat than whole milk. Whole milk already is 97 percent fat-free. Whole milk contains three percent fat, in other words. The one to two percent fat differences between low fat and whole milk, however, are significant. Using skim milk painlessly cuts calories and saturated fat from your diet. Skim milk has no fat.

To recap, then: There are several ways to make the principles of the Palm Beach Diet really work for you. *The first is to choose foods which are low in sodium and in cholesterol.* While it's true that some individuals appear less sensitive to sodium and better able to handle cholesterol, why take chances? Especially at fifty or more.

I've also suggested that the term "natural" can be deceiving—freshness or lack of processing or refining may be better clues to the quality of food. Remember that as you shop. Peruse the chart of food additives, too, to familiarize yourself with those considered safe, and those substances you'll want to avoid in excess amounts.

Finally, don't be swayed by the tricks and traps of food marketing. And store and cook your healthy foods to the best advantage. Overall, you're right on target if you choose the sort of foods that make the honor roll in Chapter 12, buy them as fresh as possible and use them as soon as possible.

CHAPTER 14

Fifty-Plus Exercise

The mere thought of exercise makes many adults want to draw the blinds and go back to bed. Many older men find exercise a needling reminder that they're no longer thirty-nine and holding, for example. At the annual office picnic, they may get coaxed into a softball game—and develop a leg cramp on the way to the plate. Senior golfers grumble that they've lost distance off the tee. Women in their fifties and sixties, meanwhile, grew up on Saturday matinees and cherry colas, not sports and exercise. The world of aerobics and "workouts" is a foreign one indeed.

Yet we know that the fifty-plus age group can perhaps benefit the most from physical activity. Exercise fights overweight, helps prevent illness and can even slow the rate of aging—all prime concerns at the prime of life.

Exercise is as important to you, now, as diet. It is as helpful to weight loss as dieting, in many cases. Some people who diet find the pounds aren't dropping at a satisfying pace—until they start exercising, too. There's a medical explanation for this: Dieting tends to lower the metabolic rate—that is, the rate at which the body burns calories. As you eat less, you need less, too. Weight loss then becomes slow and arduous. Regular exercise, on the other hand, *increases* the metabolic rate: Your peppier system continues to burn calories at an accelerated rate for some time after exercising. This phenomenon, while temporary, speeds weight loss.

Together, a good diet and exercise are the best investments you can make in yourself. They're a weight-loss team. This marriage also does more to promote longevity and good health than anything medicine has to offer!

Many people regard exercise as a sort of health "frill"—a welcome boost to the body, but something that isn't essential to health. They hear and read about the benefits of exercise—but then rationalize that they can live well without it, too. This simply isn't the case: Especially as one grows older, some physical deterioration associated with lack of exercise is nearly inevitable.

If you could "play" doctor for one day, the importance of exercise would come driving home to you. Take the exercise histories of vital, spry eighty-year-olds and compare them to the exercise histories of incapacitated eighty-year-olds, and you would almost certainly spot a trend. Regular movement—on an every day or every other day basis—prolongs and improves the quality of life.

"Okay, okay," I can hear you say. "I've heard it all before. But just look at me. I'm so out of shape, I don't know where to begin. Besides, the whole idea of exercise bores me to tears."

My response: Then reinvent your notion of exercise. Drop unrealistic expectations, and deal with the boredom factor first—the two common exercise complaints among people fifty or more.

Unrealistic expectations first. Today's booming interest in exercise makes many nonathletes feel damned if they don't join in, and yet frightened at the prospect of putting on exercise gear and overextending themselves. The whole idea of exercise can be intimidating. In recent years, the measure of a physically fit man seems to be the number of miles he can marathon. And women are made to feel like third-string rookies if they can't perform a straight hour of aerobic dance exercises.

To someone whose idea of exercise is climbing a flight of stairs, these physical fitness expectations are certainly unrealistic. Once more, they can be potentially health-damaging. And, to top it off, they're unnecessary.

Now the good news. Exercise physiologists tell us that *exercise does not have to be tiresome or exhausting to be beneficial. It does not have to be fast. It does not have to hurt. What is important is that it be sustained. Slow and steady are the by-words here. Exercise duration is more important than exercise exertion.*

Certainly it would be nice to see every healthy sixty-year-old joining in "fun runs," or keeping pace with the flash dancers in a flex class. To maintain or improve physical fitness, though, you needn't go to these extremes.

Compare the benefits of walking vs. jogging, for instance. It's true that jogging will improve heart and lung capacity faster than walking—but walking at a brisk pace improves both, too. You get similar muscle-toning rewards from each, and yet walking is less jarring, and therefore, carries lower risk of injury, than jogging. Once more, *you burn as many calories walking a mile as jogging a mile.* It just takes you longer to get there, is all.

Then there's the boredom factor. Many people find jogging tedious. Ditto for many other exercise regimens, such as jumping rope or riding a stationary bicycle: How many people, for instance, do you know who *really* use a stationary bicycle regularly and with relish?

Walking is another proposition altogether. You can enjoy the view, meet and greet neighbors, and mull whatever is on your mind at the moment. Walking is exercise "in disguise," in a way: No one has to know you're exercising. You don't need a special wardrobe; you don't have to feel self-conscious about being a beginner and "looking silly." You already know how to walk, and while you're out enjoying, something else is happening: You're reaping all the benefits I'm about to describe.

Exercise: An Antiaging Tool

Regular exercise slows the aging process, pure and simple. It does so in a number of ways.

One marker of aging, for example, is a natural loss of muscle. In many people, the muscle that is lost with age is replaced by fat. This fit-for-flab exchange is not inevitable, however; it is a function of lack of exercise, coupled with a fatty diet. A good diet, supplemented with regular exercise, can maintain and even improve muscle tone.

Another way in which movement slows the aging process has to do with blood circulation. Exercise improves blood flow to the entire body, from the cells of your brain to the cells of your big toes. Improved blood flow, in turn, helps to deliver oxygen and nutrients to cells for optimal functioning. This can improve everything from skin tone to "internal" fitness. Improved blood flow to the kidneys, for example, can slow the degeneration of the kidneys that can occur with aging.

Movement moves the inner you, too. Regular exercise helps to relieve constipation. It aids digestion as well: People who exercise regularly report fewer problems with indigestion than do sedentary sorts. Both constipation and indigestion are common complaints among people who are fifty or more.

Exercise also can act as a preventive measure against certain illnesses. It can help relieve the symptoms of other conditions. Let me give you a few examples.

There are volumes of evidence that exercise can decrease the risk of heart attack. This research into the cardiovascular benefits of exercise is generating enormous interest now. While more studies are still being done, we can already build a convincing case that endurance-type exercise, done regularly, helps maintain heart health. Regular exercise helps lower blood levels of the fatty substances *triglycerides,* it increases the levels of the heart-protective cholesterol called *high-density lipoprotein* (*HDL*) *cholesterol.* And while the case isn't nailed shut, there is evidence that regular exercise helps lower blood levels of the harmful *low-density lipoprotein* (*LDL*) *cholesterol.* Another theory is that regular endurance-type exercise may improve heart and lung function to the point of compensating for existing and partial arterial blockage. In other words, regular exercise may not prevent hardening of the arteries, but may make existing artery disease less of a factor in heart attack risk.

Diabetics are often told to get out and start moving, too. Diabetics who exercise regularly have better control of their blood sugar. Exercise makes cells more receptive to insulin, and it stimulates the body to produce more of needed insulin. Diabetics who exercise, however, must plan insulin doses carefully.

Exercise can also help you walk away from the condition known as *osteoporosis,* the wasting of bone that occurs in later life in most people. Exercise in which you bear weight on bone *strengthens* bone, and helps to counteract the loss of bone density. A regular walking or jogging program, for example, can help prevent the bone degeneration of the spine, hips and legs. (On the other hand, swimming—another top-drawer exercise—in which the body is supported by water, is of little help.)

There's plenty more if you still need convincing. Exercise physiologists theorize that regular exercise raises the levels of hormone-like substances in the brain called *endorphins.* Endorphins are natural opiate-like compounds: They appear to be the hormonal secretions that bring on a feeling of well-being. Endorphins may be responsible for the sparkling "high" that athletes claim to experience. It may be endorphins "pulling the strings" in part, too, in people who report that exercise counteracts depression.

Another exercise-boon to the mature individual is *relaxation,* believe it or not. People who begin to exercise regularly report that they sleep better for it. During waking hours they feel freer from tension.

A final consideration: When you extend your physical capability through exercise, you may become better able to cope with those curve balls life throws each of us—physical stress and personal crises. While no study proves this absolutely, it does often seem that physical well-being in the mature years promotes emotional equanimity, too.

Low-Intensity Endurance Exercise: Your Bonfire for Fat

The best-known "plus" of exercise is weight loss: Everyone knows that exercise requires energy, as measured in calories. What is less well-known is that the length of time spent exercising determines the "fuel" being used to power your movement. *After twenty to thirty minutes of continuous exercise, the body burns more fat than glycogen—the sugar "fuel" it stores and then uses for short bursts of activity.*

Once the body uses up ready energy stores, in other words, it turns to stored fat to power your movement. Hip hooray—or should I say hips good-bye! To tap into fat stores, *duration* of exercise is more important than exertion.

You can look at duration and exertion as two key variables in exercise. The most demanding combination of the two is all-out exertion over a long stretch of time—foot-racing over ten miles, for example. That's an improbable feat for most people who are fifty or more: Cutting back on one of the two variables is more realistic.

So now you have a choice. You can choose intense activity over a short period of time (running half a mile, say) or a low-intensity activity for a longer period of time (walking three miles, for example). What's the better choice if you want to lose weight *and* gain health benefits? *Low*-intensity, long-term movement on both counts.

A quick "go" at strenuous exercise will not take you over the twenty to thirty minute minimum required to begin burning more fat than glycogen as fuel, for instance. Short bursts of all-out exertion can be health-endangering, too. Sudden and intense exertion shocks the system. It raises blood pressure and is potentially dangerous to the heart. Once more, quick clips of high-intensity activity do *nothing* to improve heart and lung condition. Three strikes—and quick, all-out exercise is out!

Isn't it nice to know that a long walk is more health-supportive and slimming than a quick jog? I must emphasize "brisk," though—you must feel you're doing a little work in order to condition heart and lungs. After a warm-up period that prepares your heart, lungs and muscles for it, you must have a period of aerobic exercise in which you are aware of a faster heart and breathing rate in order to achieve fitness. A cool-down period in which your body readjusts gradually should follow. The warm-up reduces the risk of injury; the cool-down adjusts the body gradually to stopping the aerobic exercise. You should *never* be totally exhausted or out of breath. The biggest mistake I see people make is doing too much too soon. This will hurt rather than help you. Get your doctor's okay first, too.

What else should your exercise choice take into consideration? How about heart health? Dr. Ralph Paffenbarger, an epidemiologist and exercise researcher at Stanford University, believes, based on his studies of longshoremen and Harvard alumni, that exercise is associated with reduced risk of heart attack, despite the fact that relevant studies are not all in agreement. This cardiovascular "training effect" of exercise has been studied further since, and experts recommend expenditures of about 300 calories per exercise session, at least three times per week, to maintain or improve cardiovascular fitness. That's a tall order for a sedentary and overweight person of fifty or more—but not out of reach, as I'll describe in a moment.

What else counts in exercise? Accessibility. Painlessness. Enjoyment. And for those people who fear exercise—safety. And for those who cringe at the thought of getting caught in gym shorts—anonymity!

What we have, then, as parameters of exercise: safety, enjoyment, privacy. Something that is of medium intensity, but of substantial duration. Something that eventually could burn roughly 300 calories per session and thereby help protect heart health—once you've built up to training-effect levels. What fits this description? Two of Palm Beach's favorite outdoor pastimes—walking and water exercises—will do nicely.

Let's build the case for walking first:

1. A walking program will help maintain or build leg and back muscles and slow muscle loss that naturally occurs with aging.

2. A brisk walking program can help protect the heart, and deliver antiaging benefits to other parts of the body—skin, lungs and vital organs.

3. Walking a mile briskly burns as many calories as jogging a mile.

4. Any exercise (including brisk walking) performed steadily for at least twenty to thirty minutes will begin to burn more fat than glycogen for fuel.

That's an attractive list of benefits—and all you have to do is *walk*. So how do you start? Slowly. I cannot emphasize enough the importance of starting slowly if you have been inactive for a long time. Almost everyone can benefit from a walking program, but begin your walks by tackling no more than fifteen-minute sessions if you have not exercised regularly all along. Begin with five minutes of leisurely strolling, up your pace the following five minutes to a brisker walk and then cool-down to a leisurely stroll again for an additional five minutes.

Starting slowly in this manner, you will gradually build stamina. If that much is easy for you, begin to add two–three minutes more of brisk walking your second week out. Continue to add two–three minutes more of brisk walking each week—always beginning and ending with five minutes of relaxed strolling. If any week is particularly hard, repeat it—don't force yourself to do more than you feel comfortable doing. See your doctor if at any point pain, dizziness or shortness of breath results from exercise.

Eventually, you may well be able to engage in forty-five minutes of brisk walking. A brisk forty-five minute walk three to four times a week should be enough to maintain a level of cardiovascular fitness that is heart-protective. I feel a person should start with a fifteen minute warm-up; forty-five minutes aerobic brisk walk and a fifteen minute cool-down.

Of course, not everyone is ready for even fifteen minutes of out and about. If, for example, you only feel comfortable walking five minutes at first, do so and do no more—you still will benefit to some degree. Then, too, some people have difficulty walking: Those who suffer from arthritis and osteoporosis are examples. In either case, gentle exercise in a warm pool is a good alternative. Mind you, pool exercise can't cure arthritis, but it does offer relief temporarily, and can improve overall fitness. If you choose exercise in the pool, you might want to use a kick board to build up leg strength and then start with the backstroke or gentle breaststroke one pool length until you gradually build up endurance. Swimming vigorous laps is best reserved for persons already adapted to that type of training.

Other people fifty or more may be recuperating from illness, or heart attack. In either case, following your doctor's recommendation and starting *more* slowly are essential. If you get doctor-clearance, start by walking only a comfortable distance. Don't be discouraged if that's only a matter of yards or minutes: Regardless of how little you do, your fitness level is almost sure to improve gradually and satisfyingly if you stay with it. Perhaps the only advantage to being out of shape is that stamina can double or triple, with very little effort, within weeks.

This sort of gentle exercise program, by the way, is being adopted by hospitals. Heart attack recovery patients are walking to mend their hearts. Most doctors now believe that the benefits of mild, controlled exercise outweigh the cardiovascular risks of *not* exercising.

> **Palm Beach Postscript:** If you're fifty or more, and especially if you're recovering from a heart attack, you must check with your doctor before starting an exercise program. Every case is individual: Extenuating circumstances in a particular case could mandate bed rest, for example. If your doctor has advised you that you have high blood pressure or are at risk of a heart attack, check with her or him before starting any new exercise program.

More Exercise Know-How

Be sure to have a checkup if any of the following apply to you: You're over fifty, haven't exercised in a long time, have high blood pressure, a heart condition, diabetes or if you smoke heavily. You *must* have a physical examination before beginning this or any exercise program. Your doctor may also recommend a stress EKG test. The checkup and a fitness or "stress" test will help determine how much exercise you can handle safely.

If you don't feel that your family doctor, general practitioner or internist is equipped to check you thoroughly for exercise fitness, you can call your local chapter of the American Heart Association or the cardiovascular department of a local hospital for a referral. Indicate that you want to start an exercise program, are fifty or over, and hope you might be referred to a doctor accustomed to assessing physical fitness, particularly for your age group. Your prudence and motivation will surely be well-received! *Having a checkup, then, is vital preparation for exercise.*

Once you're cleared for exercise, you're ready to roll. If you haven't exercised in years, you may need a few helpful hints. Many of these are especially important tips for people fifty or more.

1. Wear loose clothes and comfortable shoes. If your clothing restricts or chafes, you won't enjoy what you're doing. A good pair of sneakers will help prevent pulled muscles.

2. Warm up with stretches before you begin. Exercise pros know you can't head into exercise "cold." To do so invites strains and pulls; it also puts sudden pressure on your heart. At fifty or more, you don't want to invite either! Warming up is the logical extension of the one exercise maxim you need remember: *Start slowly and proceed at a comfortable pace.*

Should you stretch even before walking? You should. Walking offers many physical and mental benefits, but flexibility, unfortunately, isn't among them. To keep muscles and joints loose and limber, you need to stretch. I suggest doing gentle floor exercises before you go out for your walk. Start with a minute or two of stretching overhead, side to side, and down toward your toes. Work up gradually to fifteen-minute sessions. Eventually, a fifteen-minute "stretch session" every day will help relieve muscular tension, loosen joints, improve circulation and limberness, reduce your risk of incurring arthritis and reduce your chances of injury during other exercises and sports. And calf-muscle stretches will help prevent leg cramps.

To stretch, you move all the joints of your body through their range of motion, slowly and evenly, without forcing or bouncing. Don't expect to touch your toes, for instance, if you haven't been able to do so in years. *Don't* force or bounce. By gently and steadily stretching, you will find you can go further without *having* to force. Follow these diagrams and directions if you haven't developed a stretching routine of your own. Take several deep breaths at intervals throughout the session.

Start your flexibility stretches with the ten exercises illustrated here. Do each slowly, and stretch only to the point at which you feel comfortable. Stretch smoothly; don't jerk or bounce. Ready? Here you go!

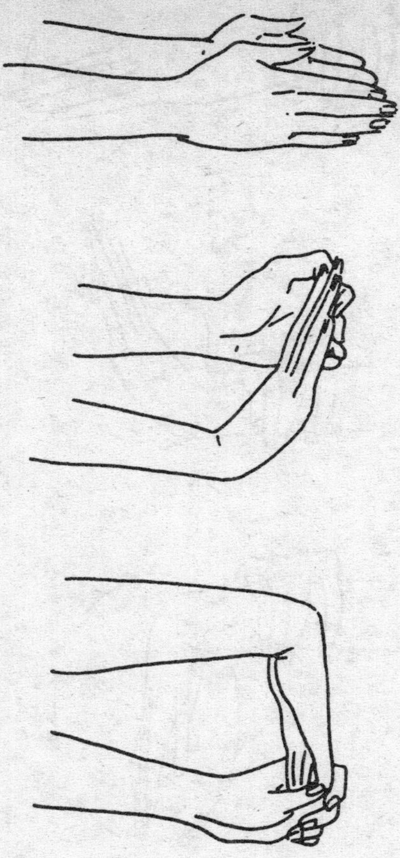

1. Finger Stretching: *to maintain finger dexterity.* With the palm of the right hand facing down, gently force fingers back toward forearm, using left hand for leverage; then place left hand on top and force fingers down. Suggested repetitions: 5 each hand.

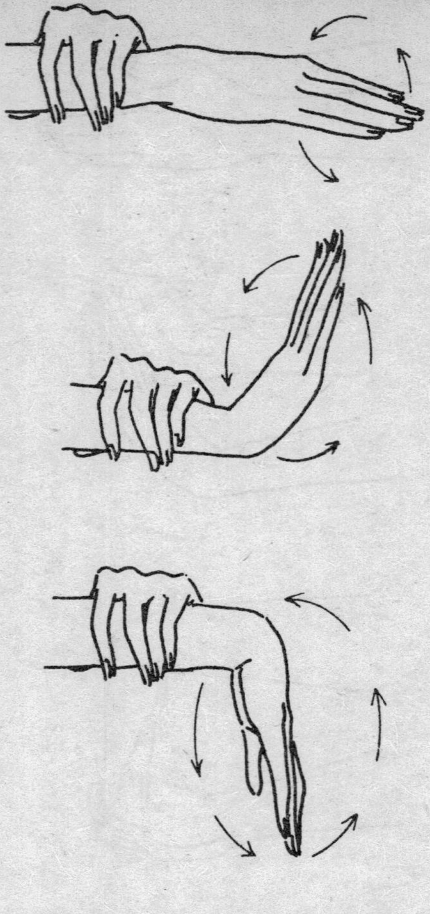

2. Hand Rotation: *to maintain wrist flexibility and range of motion.* Grasp right wrist with left hand. Keep right palm facing down. Slowly rotate hand 5 times each clockwise and counter-clockwise. Suggested repetitions: 5 each hand.

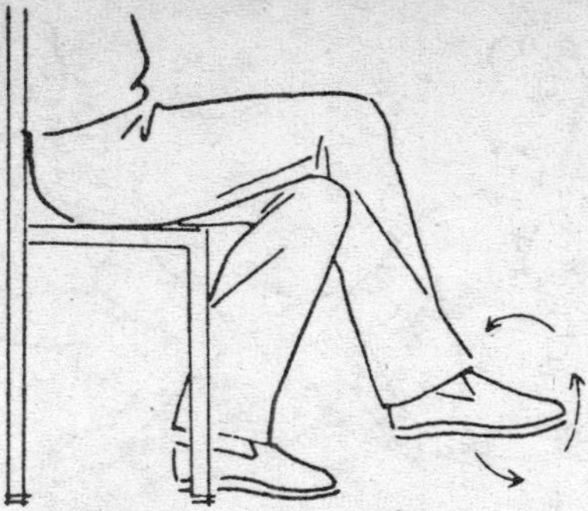

3. Ankle and Foot Circling: *to improve flexibility and range of motion of ankles.* Cross right leg over opposite knee, rotate foot slowly, making large complete circles. 10 rotations to the right, 10 to the left, each leg.

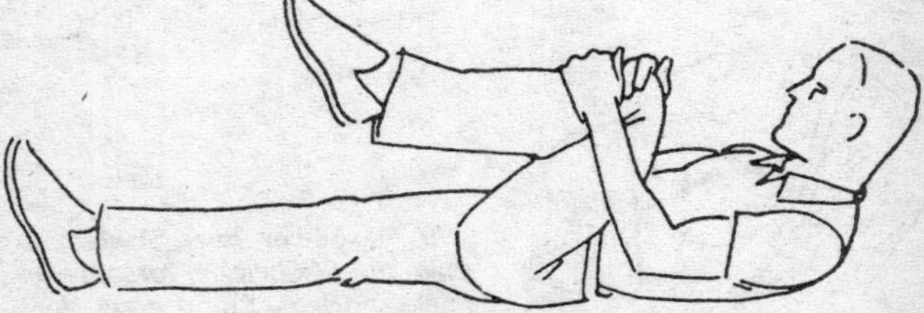

4. Single Knee Pull: *to stretch lower back and back of leg.* Lie on back, hands at sides. Pull one leg to chest, grasp with both arms and hold for five counts. Repeat with opposite leg. Suggested repetitions: 3–5.

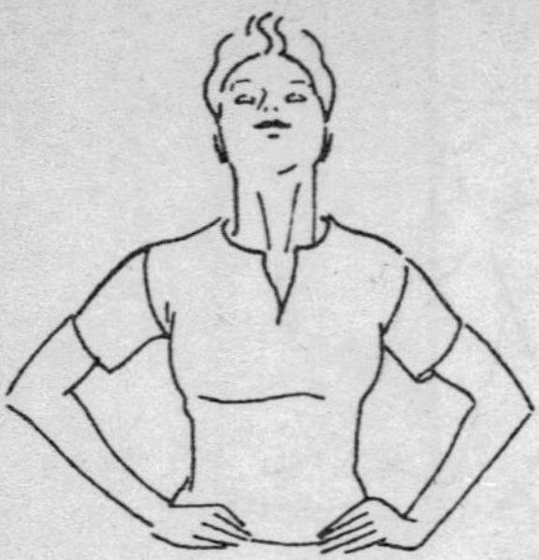

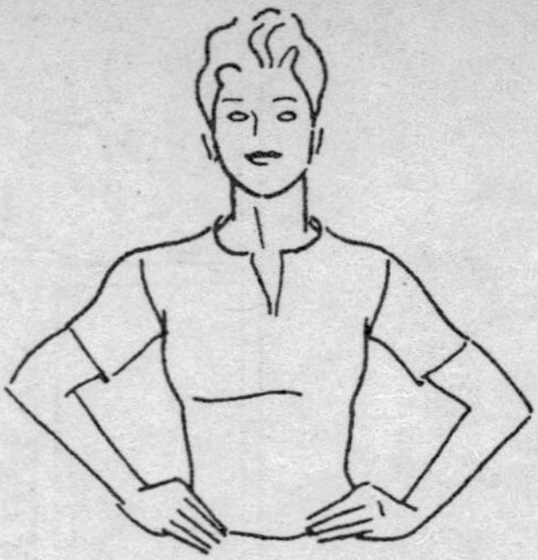

5. Neck Extension: *to improve flexibility and range of motion of neck.* Sit up comfortably. Bend head forward until chin touches chest, then bend it backward as far as it is comfortable (as shown in drawing). Return to starting position and slowly rotate head to left. Return to starting position and slowly rotate head to right (as shown in drawing). Return to starting position. Suggested repetitions: 5.

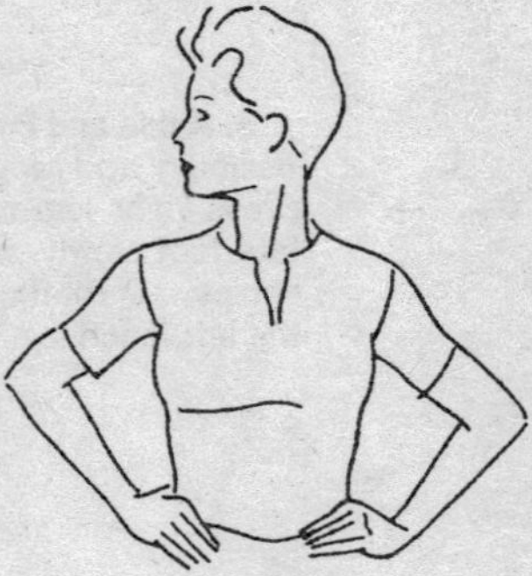

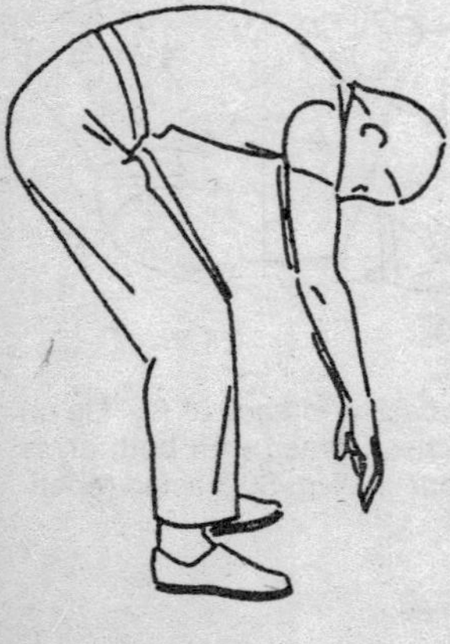

6. Flexed-Leg Back Stretch: *to maintain flexibility in torso, lower back and legs.* Stand erect, feet shoulder-width apart, arms at sides. Slowly bend forward as far as possible, preferably until you touch ground. Keep knees flexed. Hold for 10 to 15 counts. Suggested repetitions: 4–6.

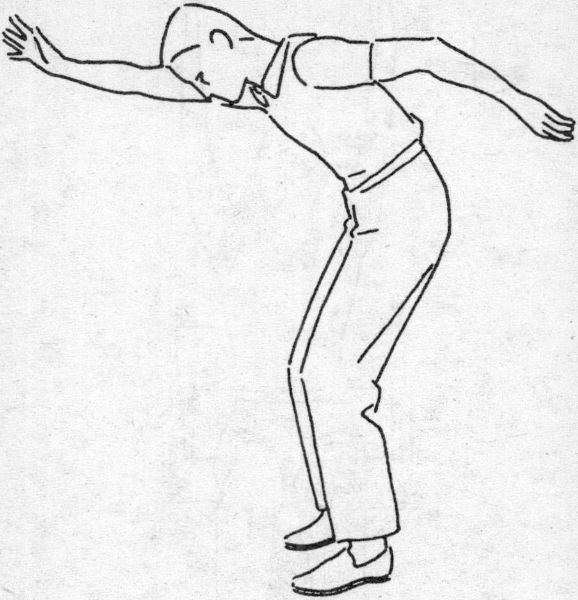

7. Simulated Crawlstroke/Backstroke/Breaststroke: *to stretch shoulder girdle.* Stand with feet shoulder-width apart, arms at sides relaxed. Bend knees and alternately swing right and left arms backward . . . upward . . . and forward as if swimming. Suggested repetitions: 6–8 movements on each stroke.

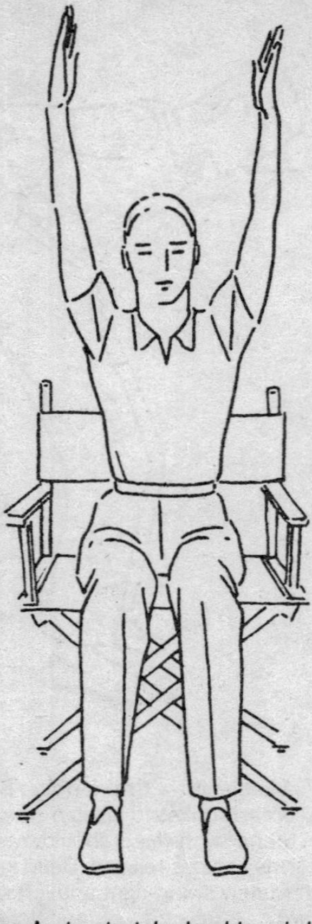

8. Reach: *to stretch shoulder girdle and rib cage.* Take deep breath, extend arms overhead. If standing, rise on toes while reaching. Exhale slowly, dropping arms. Can be done in a seated position. Suggested repetitions: 6–8.

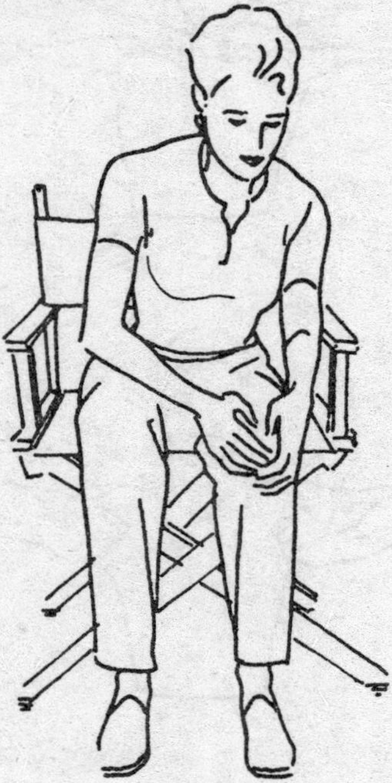

9. Backstretch: *to improve the flexibility of the lower back.* Sit up straight. Bend far forward and straighten up. Repeat, clasping hands on left knee. Repeat, clasping hands on right knee. Exhale while bending forward. Suggested repetitions: 4–6 over each knee.

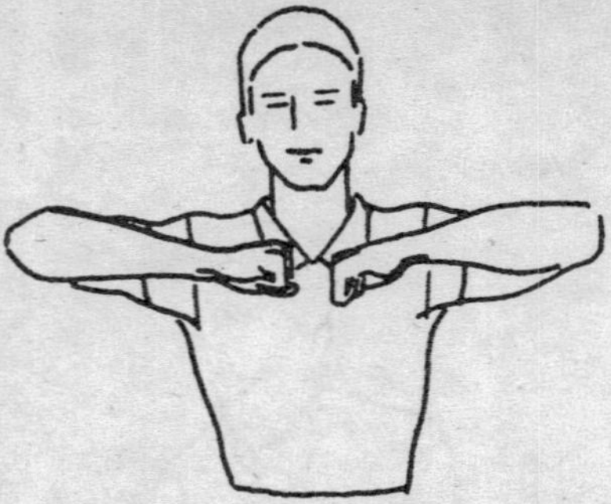

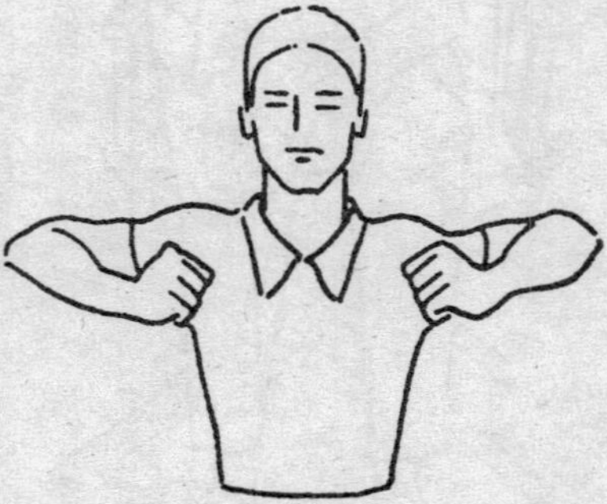

10. Chain Breaker: *to stretch chest muscles.* Stand erect, feet about 6 inches apart. Tighten leg muscles, tighten stomach by drawing it in, shove hips forward, extend chest, bring arms up with clenched fists chest high, take deep breath, let it out slowly. Slowly pull arms back as far as possible keeping elbows chest high. Suggested repetitions: 8–10.

3. Get out and walk. You should warm up fifteen minutes, walk briskly for forty-five minutes, and cool down by walking slowly for fifteen minutes. You should build up to it gradually, starting with about ten minutes the first time. Walk at least three times a week, and a walk a day is even better of course.

If you can't walk without pain—in the case of arthritis or osteoporosis, for example—gentle exercise in a warm pool is an alternative. Water exercises are especially good for you: You can spend hours in a warm pool and feel no pain. Just remember to make it a *warm* pool: Cold water is a jolt to the system. Many communities, YMCAs and YWCAs maintain a heated swimming pool. And summer swimming in tepid lakes, ocean or swimming pools is fine. If you're not a swimmer, of course, stay at the shallow end of the pool!

If you're a joiner, not a loner, a number of organizations sponsor exercise programs for nonathletes, or people with health conditions which benefit from regular exercise. Many hospitals, for example, have recently initiated cardiac fitness programs. Most are aimed at people fifty and over with preexisting health conditions such as high blood pressure, coronary heart disease, and overweight. In some cases, health insurance covers the cost of these new and burgeoning hospital exercise programs. Call your local hospital for more information. You can also find intelligently run exercise programs for nonathletes at many YMCAs and YWCAs. Your local chapter of the American Heart Association, or your public health department, may also sponsor or recommend responsible programs of preventive exercise.

4. Another exercise maxim: If you feel pain, stop. The idea that exercise should be painful to be beneficial is nonsense—especially for people fifty or more. Pain, nausea, dizziness or shortness of breath are signs that you've pushed harder than you should have. Don't play the hero or heroine: Do only what feels comfortable. With regular and gentle exercise, your body will become capable of handling more exercise with less effort.

5. Don't exercise right after eating. Wait thirty minutes to an hour after eating before taking your walk or swim. Why? When you eat a meal, a lot of blood is diverted to the intestines. If you also begin to exercise, the heart has to work hard to pump blood from the intestines to the "exercising" parts of the body. That's a strain on the heart.

By the way, it's folklore fiddle-faddle that swimming after eating will give you stomach cramps and make you sink. True, you shouldn't swim after eating, but because of the extra burden on the heart, not for fear of cramps.

6. Don't exercise in the heat of the day. It's a bad idea to take even a stroll at noon in August—especially in semitropical climates. Heat stroke can result. In summer, or in a warm climate, exercise in the early morning or at dusk.

7. Don't stop abruptly after exercising. Don't go out for a jog, for example, and brake to a halt at your front door. Slow down gradually, bringing the jog to a walk and then to a stroll. The reason: When you exercise, blood pumps briskly. Stop suddenly and blood in the lower extremities doesn't have the "oomph" to return to the heart. It may pool in the feet and legs. That can cause feelings of faintness, since less blood is now available to the brain.

8. Have a glass of water after exercising. Even if you don't feel sweaty or see perspiration, you lose water through invisible perspiration during even gentle exercise.

9. Take warm—not hot—showers directly after exercising. It may feel good to climb into a hot shower after your walk or swim, but I recommend that you turn back the temperature a little. Immediately after exercising, your blood supply still is needed by the heart muscle: Your heart needs blood now to get the oxygen it needs to work optimally. Taking a hot shower interferes with this natural dynamic: It draws blood out to the skin. Take a warm shower after you've cooled down.

Remember this as you start your exercise program: The well-being that exercise generates can become a positive addiction! You'll come to know what it is to feel sparkling and full of life—just like a kid again. You'll love it—I can almost guarantee it. Check with your doctor first, start slowly and build to longer sessions gradually, and you're on the "feel-good" road to fitness and improved health.

CHAPTER 15

Sex, and a Note on Stress

Many young people assume that older people are no longer interested in sex. Perhaps you once assumed as much of *your* older relatives and acquaintances. No doubt reality has debunked this myth for you: Sex can be as healthy and fulfilling now as it ever has been. In fact, given more experience, fewer social pressures, freedom from guilt and worries about pregnancy, mature sexual relationships can be especially gratifying.

Research in human sexuality confirms that sexual interest and activity can continue normally throughout life: Many people in their eighties and nineties are still sexually active. Certainly, intercourse may be less vigorous and less frequent, but it may last longer and improve in quality. In fact, the hardiest and healthiest eighty-year-olds and ninety-year-olds often have the twinkle in their eye of a fulfilling sexual relationship.

The context of sex can change with age—and for the better. Wisdom, tenderness, patience and history—the stuff that makes up mature emotion and underpins genuine love—enrich sexual expression.

Sex over Fifty

Until recently, what we knew of sexual attitudes and practices among Americans over fifty was largely anecdotal. Few studies undertook a methodical examination of sexuality in the mature years. Now that maturity has come of age, however, this biosocial frontier is being surveyed. For example, a fascinating report on sexual attitudes and activities of people over fifty was published in 1984 by Edward M. Brecher and the editors of Consumer Reports Books. Titled *Love, Sex, and Aging* (Little, Brown and Company), the study's findings are, in the word of the report, "astonishing." Among the findings:

- Today's grandmothers and grandfathers are notably different from *their* grandmothers and grandfathers. They are also notably different from what they themselves were like in their youth; for example, they are now sexually much freer.

- Of the 4,246 respondents to the Consumer Reports survey, 80 percent of wives and 77 percent of husbands (all over fifty) report that they are currently having marital intercourse. These husbands and wives are far more likely to report happy marriages than wives and husbands who are not having sexual intercourse with their spouse.

- While marital happiness is closely linked with "having sex with spouse" and "enjoying sex with spouse," it is less closely linked to "frequency of sex with spouse." Neither is "ease of sexual arousal" a predictor of marital happiness—for men. Women who report that they become sexually aroused with difficulty, or not at all, are more likely to report an unhappy marriage.

• There is a decade-by-decade decline in sexual activity. However, this decline is, according to the Consumer Reports survey, "an aging rather than a health effect for both men and women."

These findings may be skewed slightly, at the authors' admission, by the fact that the study subjects were drawn voluntarily from the pool of readers of Consumer Reports. The respondents would tend to have higher-than-average income and education, better-than-average health and greater interest in sex. Nonetheless, the survey findings reflect an unabashed and generally joyous attitude toward shared sexual activity in later life.

As a doctor, I find that the fear of reduced sexual ability with age often is a paper tiger. My mature patients may growl that "my sexual response isn't what it used to be"—but in fact it still remains quite normal. In fact, a frequently cited stumbling block to continued sexual enjoyment in later life isn't loss of sexual response or ill health, but lack of a suitable partner. Sexual isolation frustrates widows, widowers, singles, and people whose marriage partner isn't interested in sex. Reciprocity is a keynote of satisfying relationships: Having a willing and caring partner, it seems, is more important than objective measures of performance as we grow older. As long as neither partner demands youthful zest, or watches the clock, love-making can remain satisfying and life-affirming, regardless of age.

To those people who fear they'll lose their sexual prowess as they grow older, I have three words of advice: Don't stop now! There *is* truth to that graphic slogan "Use it or lose it." People who wish to remain sexually active into a ripe old age should avoid prolonged periods of sexual abstinence; by "prolonged period," I mean six months or more. The reason: Sexual stimulation increases the secretion of sex hormones, which in turn maintains or increases sex drive. This holds true for both men and women.

Good health isn't a prerequisite of a good sex life—but it's a big help. If a mature man is out of shape, and perhaps suffers from a health condition or two, he may feel, and therefore become, less virile. Putting on weight can undermine a woman's sense of sexual attractiveness, too. Weight loss and regular exercise to improve physical condition can be a tremendous boost to the libido in such cases. Whatever the age, body confidence is often echoed in sexual confidence. And perhaps you've noticed, too, that this works the other way around as well: Rekindled sexual interest is a spur to weight loss. How many times have you seen friends fall in love, and proceed to lose weight and look like a million again?

There are physiological reasons for lowered sexual interest, too. In men, erection may take longer to achieve, for example. For both men and women, orgasms may become less intense with age. Fortunately, most mature individuals adjust to these facts of life. They relax and enjoy.

Medications also can meddle with sexual functioning. Mood-altering drugs, including antidepressants and tranquilizers, can reduce sexual desire. The same is true of some medications prescribed for high blood pressure. Occasionally, switching to another medication can alleviate the problem. Lowering the dosage, if possible, can help. And weight loss, coupled with regular exercise, can reduce the *need* for blood pressure medicines in some cases. Don't go off prescribed blood pressure medication without your doctor's okay, of course: Check with your doctor *after* you've lost weight. Your medication dosage can perhaps be lowered at that point.

For most mature individuals, however, sexual interest and ability needn't suffer significantly just because a birthday or two has rolled by. Take inspiration from the Consumer Reports Study: Today's aging Americans seem to be growing younger—and lustier—at heart.

A Note on Stress

You may have picked up on a common thread woven throughout these chapters. Whether the subject is diet, exercise or sex, I've urged you to relax and enjoy. Don't hope, for example, to lose fifteen pounds over a weekend. Doing so can undermine your health and encourage weight rebound. Don't launch into a do-or-die jogging program if you haven't exercised in years: Start slowly—at a *walk*. Don't get "uptight" over sexual concerns: Relax and enjoy. What's the hurry?

Time urgency is a tremendous stress. The pressure of performing to the clock or to the calendar creates tension, and can aggravate illness.

Stress is the body's chemical/physical/emotional response to threats and challenges, crises and expectations. This adaption of the body to danger is a splendid survival mechanism: By pumping up your blood pressure, your heart rate and your output of adrenaline, stress can save your life in an emergency situation—having to dodge out of the way of a speeding car, for example.

Stress can also make everyday living a physiological melodrama, however. The human body responds to the small frazzles and frustrations of everyday life in much the same way it responds to the threat of danger. When there's not enough time in the day, when your sister falls ill, when you feel lonely or unappreciated or when you chastise yourself for having deviated from your diet, you may become distressed. A host of physical symptoms can result from chronic low-grade stress—symptoms such as nervousnes, irritability, tension headaches, constipation or diarrhea. Stress can cause or contribute to such illnesses as ulcers, heart disease and even overweight (if losing yourself in the comfort of a fattening snack becomes habit). Some researchers postulate that all illness, in fact, is aggravated by the chemical shenanigans of stress.

Obviously, stress symptoms should not be ignored. They can have medical consequences if they occur regularly. If tension makes you feel unwell, makes you lose sleep, encourages overeating, or makes you turn to alcohol or tranquilizers, don't ignore the problem. Don't rely on a pill to solve the problem.

In our fast-paced world, many people have to be taught how to relax. Unwinding has become a skill.

Perspective is a first step toward acquiring the ability to relax. I find it helpful whenever I'm rushed or frazzled to stop a moment and look at the bigger picture. I literally stop whatever I'm doing, take a deep breath and force myself to smile. This reminds me to stop taking myself so seriously. Often, we lose perspective and get "uptight" over things that are inconsequential.

I also find it helpful (and hope you might, too) to examine my self-expectations on occasion. Many of the small frustrations we experience are self-imposed.

What I call *affirmations* can help release tension. Relax, take a deep breath and repeat to yourself something positive and calming. I do this myself whenever my schedule is upended and I find myself on the run. I pause a moment, force myself to smile (that wipes away the grimace and unclenches the gritted teeth), and then repeat to myself several times the phrase, "I am calm, comfortable and serene." Affirmations of this sort can have a very positive effect.

Another stress-buster is a technique called *visualization.* How it works: Imagine a beautiful spot on a beach, or a clearing in the woods—a place where you have or could possibly feel completely at peace. I have such a place that I imagine in my mind's eye: It's a cove that I drive by on my way to and from the office. The water in the cove is clear blue; herons move among the mangroves. Palm fronds rustle in the wind. At night, in the moonlight, the gently lapping water sparkles with the iridescence of gold dust. Just thinking about this spot instills me with a sense of peace. Whenever I visualize it or drive past it, I experience the same soft wave of relaxation. You may want to choose a real or an imaginary spot that affects you this same way. If you can't imagine one, "borrow" this parcel of Palm Beach paradise!

As you put the Palm Beach Diet and its principles to work for you, acquiring a more youthful shape and renewing your vitality, I hope you remember to enjoy. Enjoy the process as well as the goal. Relax, smile, and sniff the orange blossoms along the way.

CHAPTER 16

The Bottom Line on Prevention

Diet and Disease

A diet for people fifty or more ultimately must be health-supportive. The ideal, of course, is to lose weight and *keep* your health. All of the particulars and principles—from diet to exercise and stress-reduction—that you've encountered on these pages pull you closer to this ideal.

In the final analysis, though, you may wonder to what extent a healthy lifestyle can hedge against illness. Can your diet defend you against disease? The answer is, *yes,* it can.

Research has demonstrated links between specific foods, specific eating habits and certain chronic illnesses that occur in later life. I'll present some of that evidence, as well as intriguing preliminary findings in this area of diet and disease, on the next pages. But first, before I sum up what the Palm Beach Diet *can* do for your health outlook, I want to tell you what it *cannot* do.

Fact: No diet can shield you from all health problems. The Palm Beach Diet, in other words, is not invincible armor; it is an arsenal of terrific advantages, however. Its medical goal is to help, to the extent that any diet can, prevent the mature onset of chronic disease. For some people, it can mean the difference between health and illness. For others, however, it can only hope to slow the process of chronic conditions that may have been "incubating" for months or years.

Most chronic illness begins in early-to-middle life. For example, the groundwork for such conditions as hardening of the arteries, or brittle bones, is laid in the twenties, thirties and forties. With age, these conditions or predispositions advance to disease states in some people. In this case, the Palm Beach Diet can act as a "drag" against more rapid progression of the condition.

How can nutrition help defend your health? You learned about four of the Palm Beach Diet's health advantages in earlier chapters. I'll recap them here:

1. The diet allows you to lose health-threatening weight.
2. The diet provides vitamins and minerals which are cofactors in important body functions.
3. The diet provides other substances, such as fiber and adequate liquids, that improve metabolic processes.
4. The diet balances food chemistry to your best health advantage.

But that's not all. The Palm Beach Diet also incorporates what we know of how food can help your immune system function efficiently. Hence:

5. The diet supports nutritionally the vital work of the immune system.

This last factor is an important advantage to everyone fifty or more. It's well known that immune function diminishes with age. Immune responses (such as recovery from infection, burns, surgery and stress) slow down. And viruses, bacteria, irritants and other foreign substances appear to have a better chance of "sneaking past" the body's watchdog cells.

You certainly don't want a poor diet, lacking in certain especially helpful nutrients, to compound immune system sluggishness. Even a mild iron deficiency, for example, will prevent watchdog white blood cells from doing their job. Another example: Without enough vitamin C, white blood cells are less able to detect and destroy invading substances. Yet another immune system "ace" is vitamin A: Too little of it compromises the production of infection-fighting antibodies. Zinc is also a key nutrient in immune system functioning. These are vitamins and minerals coveted by the body's defense machinery.

What does this mean to you, the dieter hoping for a little health assurance on the side? It means you want to get sufficient amounts of each of these nutrients. On the Palm Beach Diet, adequate amounts are *guaranteed.* You do not, however, need megadoses of these nutrients, in order to support immune system functions. Forgive me for grabbing my hobby horse once again, but it simply isn't true that if *some* is helpful, *more* is better. Megadoses of the nutrients featured on the Palm Beach Diet will not somehow further improve health. In fact, megadosing can boomerang: It seems that large amounts of some nutrients—such as vitamin C and vitamin E—*impair* the efficiency of white blood cells. Enough said.

Cardiovascular Disease

The relationship between heart disease and diet is direct and sometimes dire. Obesity is associated with what are called the *plasma lipids* in the circulatory system—you perhaps know them as cholesterol and triglycerides.

Higher plasma lipid concentrations, in turn, raise the risk of the cardiovascular diseases.

For years, researchers thought that dietary cholesterol, and saturated fat, for example, increased the risk of artery disease and heart attack for most age groups. I say "thought" because the case against cholesterol wasn't nailed shut. Researchers only speculated that this waxy fat deposited itself in walls of arteries, potentially blocking circulation and sometimes leading to heart attacks and strokes. Now, however, the cholesterol theory of heart disease is even stronger. A ten-year study involving thousands of middle-aged men has been completed by the National Heart, Lung and Blood Institute. The finding: A 2 percent decrease in coronary heart disease followed every 1 percent decrease in cholesterol levels. Study participants who lowered their blood cholesterol by 25 percent cut their risk of heart attack in half!

Conclusion: Cholesterol and saturated fat in the diet can be harmful. Why take a chance? Really tighten your belt when it comes to fatty meats, fatty cheeses, cream, eggs and whole milk. Processed foods containing substantial coconut oil and palm oil should be restricted, too. Liver—frequently touted as a health-food—also is very high in cholesterol. Lobster and even shrimp contain more than their share. No one suggests you never let these foods near your lips; in fact, shrimp is an occasional treat on the Palm Beach Diet. I do recommend you really rein in your appetite for them, however. While reducing cholesterol in your diet doesn't guarantee you've reduced cholesterol to a safe level (medication will be required in some cases), it cannot hurt, and it could help you.

Another pointer: Don't skimp on calcium. *In several studies, men and women given calcium supplements experienced a significant drop in blood levels of cholesterol.*

In other studies, inadequate calcium has been linked with high blood pressure. Defects in calcium metabolism have been shown in some people with high blood pressure. This relationship between calcium and blood pressure also holds when it's flip-flopped around: Many people with high blood pressure get less calcium in their diet than the norm. Further evidence of a relationship: When calcium is removed from the diet of laboratory rats, they show an increase in blood pressure.

For these and other reasons, calcium should be a cardinal diet "ingredient" for people over fifty. The Palm Beach Diet supplies 1000–1200 mg. of calcium every day.

On another front, certain types of fiber are associated with reduced cholesterol levels which can act against hardening of the arteries. The sorts of foods cited for helping to lower cholesterol, in substantial amounts, include apples which contain pectin and chick peas which contain guar gum. Have a run at them!

> **Palm Beach Postscript:** Some skeptics feel that it doesn't make sense to watch cholesterol in the diet after the age of fifty. They reason that damage to the arteries is already advanced at this point, in many cases. To which I reply, if you already have significant hardening of the arteries, you had best do whatever you can to slow down the process, rather than accelerate it. A little more damage can hurt a great deal more when you already have a partially blocked artery. It is not too late to apply preventive medicine—*as long as you don't put off getting necessary medical care in the meantime.*
>
> An interesting aside, regarding cholesterol and aging: After the age of about sixty-five, cholesterol becomes less significant a risk factor in heart disease for men. We can only speculate why this is

statistically so. I don't recommend a fatty diet, though, at any age!

High blood pressure or "hypertension" is separate from but related to heart disease. High blood pressure occurs when blood pumps through the arteries with too forceful a head of pressure, requiring the heart to work harder. *About 75 percent of all Americans have high blood pressure by the age of sixty-five.*

The relationship between high blood pressure and cardiovascular problems is direct. If you have high blood pressure and it is untreated, your odds of having a heart attack are *double to triple* those of people with normal blood pressure. The odds of having a stroke are *seven times* as great when blood pressure is high. The higher the blood pressure, the greater the health risk. High blood pressure is one of the greatest threats to the health and longevity of our population.

Most cases of high blood pressure are a mystery; the cause is unknown. Many such cases of high blood pressure can be linked, though, with an identifiable factor, such as family history, stress, alcoholism, obesity or diet. The last two causes are of concern here. They are further indictment against two popular excesses—too many calories and too much salt.

How do surplus calories, in the form of overweight, raise blood pressure? Well, one reason, believe it or not, is that the fat you put on over the holiday season, for instance, and hope to lose by springtime, doesn't just tack on to stomach, hips and thighs like a magnetic memo holder to a refrigerator door. It integrates with the body: The body grows tiny vessels called capillaries into the fat. A little added fat adds extra capillaries. That means your heart must work harder to pump blood around your extra circulatory network, resulting in higher blood pressure. This is an oversimplification, and just one of many factors, but perhaps it will give you a helpful mental picture to motivate your weight loss.

Anyone with high blood pressure therefore should maintain an ideal weight. *Weight loss can actually lower blood pressure.*

I mentioned salt, too. Most people are aware that salt raises blood pressure in some people. It does so by encouraging water retention (especially in combination with low dietary potassium); water-retention, in turn, increases the volume of fluid in the arteries, which means you have more pressure within the arteries. The heart must pump harder to get the kidneys to "unload" sodium, too.

A low-salt diet is the standard prescription for high blood pressure, along with medication, when necessary. Mind you, research has not shown that salt restriction will *prevent* high blood pressure, but it's clear that salt restriction is an important part of management of high blood pressure.

The Palm Beach Diet's double-helping advice for high blood pressure, then:

- Lose weight if you're overweight. Maintain the weight you were at 25.

- Keep salt intake down to 1–5 g. per day. Rule of thumb: You can have the occasional commercially prepared food (notoriously high in salt) but do not salt your food at the table, or add salt during cooking.

Palm Beach Postscript: The Palm Beach Diet is a low-salt diet, containing from 4–5 g. of salt per day. As it is also a weight-loss diet, it is a sound plan for the overweight person with high blood pressure. Anyone with high blood pressure should check with their doctor before starting this or any diet, however. Some cases of high blood pressure may be significant enough to require even lower salt intake than on the Palm Beach Diet. Many cases of high blood pressure require medication while the diet is being followed. If you have been prescribed blood pressure medication, continue taking it while dieting. After finishing with the weight reduction portion of the diet, you may want to check with your doctor about possibly adjusting your medication, and pursuing a low-salt maintenance diet.

If a person with high blood pressure can keep weight down, keep salt intake low, and get moderate exercise, he or she may find the requirement for blood pressure medication decreases. This is not true in all cases, however; every case of high blood pressure requires individual monitoring by a doctor.

Diet and Cancer

Some of the cancers plaguing America today can be prevented by diet. *About half of all cancers incurred in women, and about 30 percent of those contracted by men, are linked to the controllable factor of diet.* (Smoking is the leading preventable cause of cancer.)

Cancer is the second leading cause of death in America, after heart disease. For some people, the mere mention of the word sends shivers up the spine; they are reluctant to learn anything about the disease. But there is good news. A diet that combines all the known cancer-fighting nutrients, and is low in cancer-causing substances, can help prevent the disease. But the sooner you begin such a diet, the better.

There is another interesting and optimistic fact about cancer, according to analysis at the National Institute on

Aging: Cancer deaths peak at about age sixty-five, and then level off at around age eighty. Only 12 percent of deaths at age eighty are due to cancer! Perhaps all those who were going to get cancer got it, or perhaps the aging process protects against cancer in some way; the slowdown of cell division in the older system may limit or impede cell mutations, including cancers.

To understand how nutrients can battle cancers, you need to understand something about the disease itself. Cancer is the abnormal multiplication of cells. It is not simply a matter of being exposed to a cancer-causing substance and then developing the disease, however. There are a number of "actors" involved. Some can convert harmless substances into cancer-causers; others can prevent innocent chemicals from being converted into trouble-makers. My point: *The risk of cancer depends on the biochemical environment and nutritional status of the body.*

While the findings *are* controversial, one group of researchers, for example, has reported that juices prepared from cabbage, broccoli, green pepper, eggplant, apple, shallots, ginger, pineapple, and mint leaf reduced the activity of one trouble-making substance. Other investigators have found an "antimutagenic" talent in extracts of leaf lettuce, parsley, Brussels sprouts, mustard greens, spinach, cabbage, broccoli and other vegetables—all according to the report, "Diet, Nutrition and Cancer" from the National Academy of Sciences.

One of the substances which protects against changes within genes appears to be the plant pigment, chlorophyll, although other helpers within these foods also are thought to be at work. Some of these "helpers" are nutrients. Vitamin A has definite anticarcinogenic effects, for example. Vitamin E and selenium appear helpful as well.

The one "hitch" to all this good news is that the application of laboratory research—and much of the preceding *is* only laboratory research—to human immunity remains to be studied, and confirmed. A compound that prevents a chemically induced cancer from forming in the lab is not necessarily going to do the same in the human body. The body is more complex than a test tube, for better or for worse! Starting a health-inducing diet at the age of fifty is less effective than if the diet is started at age twenty or thirty. These considerations should temper over-enthusiasm, and the sort of life-extension zeal that finds disciples downing bushels of this and fistfuls of that in order to defy mortality. Preliminary findings of this sort invite us to include potentially protective foods in the diet every day; they should not lead anyone to the trough of fanaticism. No one is going to get or stay healthy subsisting only on bushels of Brussels sprouts, for instance.

The Palm Beach Diet includes one of the "antimutagenically talented" foods cited nearly every day, and often more than once a day. You find spinach in salads and with brunch eggs; broccoli as a recommended dinner vegetable; lots of fresh parsley, which is a menu-style maker as well. Throughout the diet, apple and pineapple may be your choices for the mid-morning fruit break. I want to emphasize the importance of varying your vegetable and fruit choices: To the best of our knowledge of nutrition today, *variety is more important to long-term health than the inclusion of one or two "special" foods.*

Remember that too much of a good thing makes it a bad thing. Vegetables—seemingly innocuous vegetables—included. Vegetables such as Brussels sprouts, spinach and cabbage, for instance, all contain a substance which destroys vitamin B_1. Consuming huge amounts of these vegetables raw can cause a vitamin B_1 deficiency!

Two more points before we finish our consideration of diet and cancer: One is fiber; fat is the other. You want the first, and by now you know you don't want the second.

"Bulky" fiber (in bran and vegetables, for example) is an important preventive measure against cancer of the colon. These fibers also help relieve constipation, a common complaint among people over fifty. Cancer-protection and relief of constipation, in fact, are part of the same dynamic: Fiber quickens the transit time from ingestion to elimination, which prevents cancer-causing agents from prolonged contact with the lining of the colon.

A bad actor in cancer, meanwhile, is fat. Fat is a promoter of cancer. It doesn't cause the disease itself, but it is in the supporting cast. Overweight is closely linked with cancer of the uterus. Breast, colon, ovarian and prostate cancer are associated with high-fat diets. *If you're overweight, losing weight may decrease your risk of developing these common cancers.*

Diet and Diabetes

The theme should be humming through your mind by now: Many chronic diseases associated with aging are aggravated by overweight. More than your pride should tell you to lose excess weight: I hope common sense is nudging you in the ribs by now, too.

Diet deeply influences the type of diabetes that comes on in the middle-to-mature years in people who are overweight. This type of *diabetes mellitus* generally does not require insulin injections. In many cases, it is almost completely diet-dependent. Let's take a closer look.

Diabetes is the inability of the body to produce or use insulin in response to a rise in the sugar level of the blood. It's not simply a "sugar problem," though. Diabetes also disorders protein and fat metabolism, and damages blood vessels and in turn can damage kidneys, eyes and heart. It also can damage the nervous system. Here are the facts:

- Of the 2,000,000 or so people in America with diabetes, 80 percent are over forty-five years of age.
- The peak incidence of noninsulin dependent diabetes is between the ages of fifty and seventy.
- After the age of forty, twice as many women as men develop diabetes.

Don't despair: Weight reduction and the right diet can often correct the disease. Certain types of foods can keep later-life diabetes under control, if not correct it. *Wherever grains, vegetables and cereals are the chief diet staples, diabetes is rare.*

Another nutritional factor in diabetes is *chromium.* Chromium works with insulin to help cells take in sugars. You therefore want adequate chromium in your diet, whether you are diabetic or not. All you need do to ensure your chromium "status," however, is to use whole grain breads—refined bread is stripped of some trace minerals, chromium included—and to include cheese, seafood and, occasionally, meat in your diet. Chromium concentrations in the body decrease with age: The simple act of choosing whole grain breads over white bread helps ensure your receiving enough of this important nutrient.

Palm Beach Postscript: It is foolhardy to take chromium supplements to reduce the insulin requirement of diabetes. Chromium cannot replace insulin or any of the diabetes pills.

Diet and Diverticulosis

Another health-ringer, *diverticulosis* is a condition that diet can modify or prevent. Diverticulosis is a condition in which there are diverticuli, or pouches, in the wall of the large intestine. They are caused by a low-fiber diet, which forces muscles to strain in order to move intestinal contents. The problem is common—yet rare in vegetarians and wherever the diet is high in "bulky" fiber found in bran and vegetables. In America, where vegetarianism is the exception, the fiber intake generally is low; *about half of the population over seventy have diverticulosis.*

Diverticulosis can develop into a serious condition called, not surprisingly, diverticu*litis.* It's an intestinal infection which causes pain, diarrhea and bleeding. While a high-fiber diet can slow or prevent further pouching, another tack is prescribed when the problem turns into an attack of diverticulitis. Temporarily, a low-fiber diet along with antibiotics are in order. Once the attack is controlled, a high fiber diet can be resumed.

> **Palm Beach Postscript:** Some forms of irritable bowel and colitis can be aggravated by a high-fiber diet. If you have a digestive disorder, check with your doctor before starting this or any diet.

Diet and Tooth/Gum Disease

By the age of sixty-five, one of every two Americans has lost their teeth. Among those who are sixty-four to seventy-five years of age, and still have their teeth, two-thirds have *periodontal disease*—loss of bone from the jawbone. This loss of bone mass leads to loose teeth—and then to lost teeth.

The cause of periodontal disease isn't precisely known. Some researchers speculate that an infection is the cause; others suggest that the disease is diet-related. Hormone imbalances appear to play a role.

One significant nutrient in periodontal disease is calcium. The jaw and teeth are bone, and subject to the same wasting dynamic of other bone. Some cases of periodontal disease can be viewed as osteoporosis of the jawbone, in fact. Calcium supplementation, begun before the disease is advanced, is a worthwhile preventive measure.

A less direct nutritional link with the disease is folic acid deficiency. A lack of folic acid can cause inflammation of the gums—a potential, although not an inevitable, first step toward periodontal disease.

On the Palm Beach Diet, both calcium and folic acid adequacy is assured.

On another front, tooth decay and the accumulation of bacterial plaque on teeth compound tooth and gum disease. Avoiding sugar—the dentists' rallying cry—is a strong defense against dental problems later in life. A high-fiber diet appears to help maintain teeth and gums as well: Fibrous foods stimulate the production of saliva, which contains bacteria-killers!

Diet and Osteoporosis

Osteoporosis is the wasting of bone that can result in subtle to severe disfigurement and pain. It's a prime cause of bone fractures: When bones lose density and strength, fractures can occur spontaneously. According to one survey, the condition is more than epidemic in later life among women. By the age of eighty, almost all women experience some degree of osteoporosis. The facts:

- Approximately 7 percent of fifty-year-old women have osteoporosis. Some observers believe that the incidence of osteoporosis in middle age is on the rise.

- Osteoporosis is severe enough to result in fractures in up to 30 percent of people over sixty-five.

- The female/male ratio of osteoporosis sufferers is 4:1. The disease generally occurs in men at a later age, and less severely, than it does in women.

The cause of osteoporosis remains unknown. There are clues, however. The first, and a puzzling, "actor" in osteoporosis in women is the female hormone estrogen. Most bone loss in women occurs after menopause, suggesting that estrogen somehow protects against the disease. Estrogen appears to slow the activity of cells that break down bone. Beginning at the onset of menopause, estrogen is lost—apparently increasing the rate of bone loss.

Another "mover and shaker" in osteoporosis is calcium. Bones are made of salts of calcium, phosphorus and other minerals. As a person ages, calcium loss from bones accelerates. During the first three decades of life, the body favors bone *building;* at roughly the age of fifty for women and sixty for men, the body begins favoring bone thinning. Calcium loss from bone is a key dynamic of bone thinning.

Your calcium status throughout life in part determines the density and the strength of bone going into the crucial fifth and sixth decades of life, when bone thinning occurs most rapidly. You might look at it this way: If you've had adequate calcium in your diet all along, you can "indulge" some calcium loss now, at fifty or more, without weakening bone dangerously. On the other hand, if you've avoided milk, cheese and other dairy products, have consumed plenty of meats, sodas and other phosphorus-high (and calcium-razing) foods, and also have used laxatives regularly (laxatives carry calcium and other minerals from the bowel)—you may be low in calcium. Lack of exercise can work against you here, too: Walking and jogging strengthens bone.

What to make of all this? The qualifying truth is that, once osteoporosis has developed, it cannot be reversed by diet. You can slow the rate of bone-thinning, however, by being sure to get enough calcium and regular exercise.

These are some of the specific conditions which diet and exercise can help prevent. There are no guarantees, of course—just wise and unwise choices. Throughout these pages, you've come to recognize what's best for your system, your shape and your well-being—that intangible "feel good" quality that makes living a pleasure. I sincerely hope you seriously consider the advice and feel the inspiration of the Palm Beach Diet, and make the years ahead fulfilling and sparkling.

Appendix

Medications, Drugs and Diet

The American over fifty who does not use over-the-counter medications, or take a prescription drug, is rare indeed. Most do. There are about 100,000 drugs available to people in this country. There are probably more drug choices than food choices—an interesting if disquieting observation.

The older you are, the more likely it is that you use medications, at least occasionally. And as you get older, your body does not usually handle drugs as well or as predictably. For both of these reasons, you should be familiar with the basics of drug and food interactions.

A drug is any substance used as a medicine. A number of nonprescription, or over-the-counter, items are drugs, too. You may not think of laxatives and aspirin as drugs, but they are. Even vitamins in megadose levels can have drug effects. Coffee, tea and cola contain caffeine, which is a drug. Alcohol is a drug. As you can begin to guess, there are thousands of drug interactions, and thousands of interplays between food substances and medicines.

My purpose here is to acquaint you with any "shady connections" between common food substances and common drugs—those interactions which can result in medical complications. I'll kick off with a substance sprinkled throughout these chapters—sodium.

Sodium

By now you know that too much sodium in the diet is associated with high blood pressure and fluid retention in some people. The Palm Beach Diet limits sodium to 4 or 5 g. (4000–5000 mg.) per day, for these reasons. Certain drugs, however, can propel sodium intake through the roof: They can contain huge amounts of sodium. This isn't a worry if you're in good health, and without blood pressure problems; it *is* a matter for concern if you suffer from high blood pressure, heart trouble, kidney trouble or fluid retention, however.

Most antacids, for example, contain significant to *enormous* amounts of sodium. The exceptions are the few specifically labeled "sodium free" or "does not contain salt." (The calcium carbonate antacids cited in the Palm Beach Diet are among the "no salt" antacids. Rest easy!)

Antacids which contain sodium can deliver it in great wallops! Most contain anywhere from 0.1 to 7 g. (100 mg. to 7000 mg.) of sodium. The antacid-pain reliever combinations that fizz when plunked in water generally contain from 500 to 1000 mg. of sodium per dose. Sodium bicarbonate (baking soda) is used for indigestion by many people: It also is sodium-high.

A number of laxatives and sleeping aids also contain sodium. Read package labels on nonprescription medications for sodium content. If you're not sure whether the particular medication contains more sodium than is advisable for you, check with your doctor.

Nonprescription, over-the-counter antacids, laxatives and sleeping aids which are high in sodium may counteract the effects of diuretics or water pills prescribed for fluid retention or high blood pressure. Check with your doctor before combining any of these nonprescription medications with prescribed diuretics.

By the way, one drug which should not be taken on a very *low* sodium diet is lithium, generally prescribed for depression. Lithium toxicity can develop if the body gets too little sodium. The sodium level of the Palm Beach Diet is safe—although your doctor may allow you more salt if you take lithium.

The Ins and Outs of Aspirin

The cliché "as American as apple pie" *could* be changed to "as American as aspirin." Americans consume 50 billion tablets of aspirin per year. It is a marvelous drug for fever, pain, swelling, arthritis and for discouraging the blood clotting which can lead to heart attack or stroke. And yet aspirin, if it were introduced today, probably would not be approved by the Federal Food and Drug Administration: It has many side effects and interactions. (In fact, aspirin never has been officially approved.)

Many people cannot tolerate aspirin because it causes stomach distress: It can cause gastrointestinal bleeding and iron-deficiency anemia. Ironically, this type of anemia is often treated with iron supplements, which may aggravate stomach distress further. I generally recommend that individuals who experience distress from aspirin switch to an aspirin substitute.

As I mentioned, aspirin discourages blood clotting. It does so by affecting the stickiness of the platelets needed for clotting. This anticlotting action of aspirin can affect certain drug actions. Taken together, for example, aspirin and the blood-thinning drug Coumadin can cause serious bleeding. Anyone taking Coumadin should have been told by their doctor or their pharmacist not to take aspirin. (Those people who take Coumadin also should avoid excessive amounts of foods high in vitamin K, such as liver, and go easy on leafy vegetables. Vitamin K *promotes* blood clotting, counteracting the work of the drug.)

Aspirin interferes with the body's ability to use vitamin C, too.

Anyone who takes aspirin regularly should take a 100 to 500 mg. supplement of vitamin C.

Antacids

Antacids are prescribed for ulcers and excess stomach acid. Many people also take them for everything from upset stomach to heartburn. Most are nonprescription, over-the-counter medicines. They aren't without side effects and interactions, however.

On the Palm Beach Diet, antacid tablets may be used as a calcium supplement—but only those antacid tablets which do not contain sodium or aluminum. The reason: Sodium can increase blood pressure and encourage water retention. Aluminum (often in the form of aluminum hydroxide) causes calcium to be liberated from bone, possibly encouraging weakening of bone. Antacids which contain calcium carbonate but *not* sodium or aluminum then, are the best choices for people fifty or more.

Calcium carbonate antacid tablets do interact with some vitamins, however, rendering those vitamins less available to the body. Iron, phosphorus and vitamin B_1 may be slightly compromised, although the five to six tablets a day cited in the Palm Beach Diet will not jeopardize your levels of these nutrients. No one should take more than five to six antacid tablets a day, however. Taking a lot of antacids can turn the blood dramatically and dangerously alkaline. "Megadosing" on antacids also can cause fluid retention. Don't overdo on antacids.

> **Palm Beach Postscript.** If you take antacids, check with your doctor if you have kidney disease, kidney stones, a history of hypercalcemia (high blood calcium), drink a lot of milk, take vitamin D supplements or take calcium-blocking drugs. Also check if you use theophylline, a drug used for breathing disorders. Antacids can increase the potency of the drug. Antacids should not be taken with the drug cimetidine (Tagamet is the brand name) prescribed for ulcers and other stomach conditions. Antacids can inactivate the drug.

Laxatives

Most laxatives speed up the transit time of food through the system. This can mean that you lose nutrients in the stool before they have a chance to be absorbed.

Mineral oil, for example, is a popular home remedy for constipation. Mineral oil can rob you of the fat-soluble vitamins A, D, E and K by decreasing their absorption, however. This nutrient loss can be significant: I don't recommend mineral oil as a laxative on a routine basis. Incidentally, stool softeners also compromise vitamins A, D, E and K.

Saline laxatives, such as Epsom salts, phospho-soda and magnesium citrate, can cause dehydration and deplete the body of magnesium if used frequently. Regular use should be discouraged.

Overuse of irritant laxatives, meanwhile, can cause dehydration and potassium depletion, with symptoms of fatigue muscle cramping and heartbeat irregularities. These are the laxatives which include such ingredients as "senna," "cascara," "phenolpthalein" or castor oil. Don't use any of these laxatives habitually.

Remember, many food–drug mixes are significant only over the long term, when a drug is taken regularly. This is the case with laxatives. Taking a laxative now and again will not threaten your nutritional status. Chronic use can.

Bulk-forming laxatives probably are the safest of this bunch, from a nutrition eye-view. They work much the same way that bran does—but more expensively, of course. Metamucil and Serutan are two common bulk-forming laxatives. Some of this group, however, contain sugar—not enough to add significant calories to your diet, but enough to prevent diabetics from using them in some cases. Diabetics should seek their doctor's advice on laxatives.

Enemas—yet another purgative—should be used only under a doctor's supervision. Enemas can deplete the body of minerals; they also can be habit-forming.

My preference in laxatives are bran, water, prune juice, exercise and stress reduction. You don't have to buy any of these over-the-counter; none requires a prescription.

Alcohol

Alcohol is a drug which affects the nutritional status of the body in a number of ways. It's also a nasty mixer with other drugs: About half of the hundred most frequently prescribed medicines have at least one ingredient known to interact adversely with alcohol, according to the *Harvard Medical School Health Letter*.

Mixing alcohol with tranquilizers such as Valium, Seconal or Darvon can be fatal. Many famous people have ended *bottoms up* forever for having mixed drinking and pill-popping. Alcohol exaggerates the effect of many drugs, such as epilepsy drugs, sleeping pills and some tranquilizers. Alcohol can compromise nutrients, too: Excessive drinking is a major cause of vitamin B_1 (thiamine) and folic acid deficiency. Alcohol interferes with the conversion of vitamin B_6 to its effective form, and increases the loss of zinc and magnesium from the intestines. Even the social drinker who takes two drinks before dinner is *not* immune to this alcohol-nutrient interplay.

Interactions ad nauseam

There are hundreds more possible interactions between drugs and diet. The following is the tip of an iceberg—the more common, or more serious, interactions. If you are taking one or several of these medications and have a question about drug–food mixes, query your doctor or pharmacist.

Certain diuretic and blood pressure drugs are prescribed to prevent loss of potassium. These include Aldactone, Moduretic, Dyazide and Aldactazide among others. *Never* take potassium supplements without a doctor's recommendation, especially if you take these drugs: Dangerously high blood potassium levels can result. (The potassium level of the Palm Beach Diet, or any *balanced* diet, is safe.)

To confuse matters, most diuretics cause potassium *loss.* You need adequate potassium in your diet if you use one of the many common diuretics. Your doctor probably prescribed potassium supplements along with your diuretic, if needed. Do *not* take potassium supplements on your own: Potassium levels which are too low or too high could be fatal. Check with your doctor instead.

Certain foods can make thyroid drugs less effective. People on thyroid medications should avoid excess amounts of such foods as broccoli, cauliflower, kale, kohlrabi, soybeans, Brussels sprouts, cabbage, rutabaga and turnips. If you take thyroid medication and want to follow the Palm Beach Diet, it's okay to substitute other vegetables wherever the diet calls for any of those just listed, but it's probably not necessary if you get a wide variety.

Antibiotics and diet connect, too. Different antibiotics affect different nutrients different ways. Some antibiotics kill the bacteria which produces vitamin K, for example. The antibiotic tetracycline "locks horns" with iron: Taking tetracycline with iron can decrease the absorption of tetracycline. You can avoid an interaction between the two by spacing intake of tetracycline and iron at least three hours apart. Milk and other dairy products, meanwhile, inactivate tetracycline. Avoid this combination, too. Allow at least an hour between the two.

Iron supplements, by the way, are popular with mature individuals. They're taken to combat fatigue—that "run-down feeling." Iron supplementation in excess, however, can cause poor appetite, nausea, vomiting, diarrhea or constipation, colic, gas and heartburn. Iron supplements are tricky, too: Different people tolerate different iron supplements in different ways! If you use one and experience any of the preceding symptoms, switch to another. And remember not to overdo.

By the way, coffee taken within two and a half hours of an iron supplement can lower the absorption of iron. Caffeine is the culprit: It decreases the absorption of this important nutrient. Coffee can also counteract the effects of sedatives and antianxiety drugs.

Two more drug–food interactions deserve mentioning even though the drugs involved are infrequently prescribed. The first: A group of medications called monamine oxidase inhibitors (Nardil and Parnate are brand names) taken for severe depression or high blood pressure, react with the food substance called tyramine.

Tyramine is present in a long list of foods: aged cheeses, red wine, chocolate, beer, pickled herring, figs, unrefrigerated yogurt, meat and fish, bananas, chicken liver, raisins, avocados, sour cream, yeast, and in foods prepared with meat tenderizers. These drugs, in combination with any of these foods, could raise blood pressure to critical levels

The second relatively uncommon case of interaction: Vitamin B_6 interferes with L-dopa, a drug prescribed for Parkinson's disease. People who take L-dopa should not take multivitamin supplements and foods high in vitamin B_6—as little as 10 mg. of vitamin B_6 can reverse the therapy.

How Foods Influence Drug Strength

Certain foods—and even one nutrient—can affect the dosage level of many drugs.

The principle at work here is easy to grasp: What you eat tends to affect the acidity or alkalinity of urine. Food substances such as protein, cereals, grains, cranberries, plums and prunes can cause an acid urine, for example. This acidity can increase the excretion rate, and thereby *decrease* the effectiveness of alkaline drugs, including many antidepressants, antihistamines, Quinidine for heart irregularities and theophylline for breathing. Because these drugs dissolve in an acid urine, they will work less effectively.

Other foods can create an alkaline urine, meanwhile, which tends to *decrease* alkaline drug excretion and thereby *increase* certain drug potencies. These foods include most vegetables, milk and citrus fruits. High carbohydrate diets also result in an alkaline urine.

The point to come away with is that a balanced and a varied diet, in which no one food or food group predominates, provides the optimal biochemical "milieu" for drugs. As long as you get vegetables *and* grains, for example, or dairy products *and* cereals, you needn't worry that a biochemical imbalance will affect drug dosages.

Full Stomach; Empty Stomach

You're told to take some drugs on an empty stomach: others with meals. The "with meals" recommendation is generally specified to prevent stomach upset. Medications best taken on a full stomach to decrease stomach distress include aspirin, arthritis medicines such as Motrin and Naprosyn, potassium supplements and iron supplements.

As often, you're told to take a medication on an *empty* stomach. The reason may be that the drug is absorbed better and goes to work faster and more fully when it doesn't have to compete with food in the stomach. The drug acetaminophen (Tylenol, Datril), for example, is absorbed five times faster on an empty stomach than it is after consuming a high carbohydrate meal.

Some drugs should not be taken with foods because certain foods can inactivate them. This is the case, for example, with the antibiotic tetracycline. When taken within one hour of milk or other dairy products, tetracycline is inactivated.

Most antibiotics, in fact, are best taken on an empty stomach, unless your doctor prescribes otherwise. If you eat first, the absorption of antibiotics such as penicillin and Keflex is reduced. Therefore, you may not get an adequate dose.

The following medications are also best taken on an empty stomach: Digoxin (for heart conditions), L-dopa (for Parkinsonism), and most tranquilizers and antidepressants. The reason: These drugs are absorbed in the intestines, rather than the stomach, and food prolongs the time it will take for them to reach the intestines. If these drugs are held up by food in the stomach, their effectiveness may be compromised.

In medicine, there always seems to be a special case or two. A drug prescribed for fungus infections, called griseofulvin, appears to be absorbed better if taken with a fatty meal. And vitamin B_1 supplements are best absorbed if taken with a soft drink. (On the Palm Beach Diet, however, you shouldn't need vitamin B_1 supplements, nor should you drink soda!)

Coated tablets are another case. Some medicines, such as aspirin and potassium, are available with a coating designed to bypass the stomach, and consequently cause less stomach distress. When coated capsules are taken with food, however, they are absorbed more slowly. This isn't cause for concern with potassium supplements, for example, but in the case of coated aspirin, slowed absorption means slowed pain relief. Take coated tablets on an empty stomach.

Many people are not aware that taking capsules with *ice* water slows absorption of capsule contents. Why? Because most capsule casings are made of gelatin, which dissolves more quickly in tepid or hot water. Again, this may not be crucial with some medications, but if you're taking a sleeping pill in capsule form, for instance, you want to get to sleep tonight—not tomorrow! The best way to take *any* pill, in fact, is to take a sip of water—at room temperature—then swallow the pill with water, and follow with a little more water.

FOOD AND DRUG INTERACTIONS

The following are common food and drug interactions. Some render either the involved drug or a particular nutrient less effective. If you have any doubts about how certain food substances may affect a prescribed drug, or vice versa, ask your doctor or your pharmacist for advice.

This drug:	combined with	can result in:
Acetaminophen (Tylenol, Datril)	food	slower absorption of the drug
Many antibiotics	food	slower absorption of the drug
Caffeine	iron	lowered absorption of iron
Coumadin	vitamin K	decreased effectiveness of the drug
L-Dopa	vitamin B_6	decreased effectiveness of the drug
Tagamet	iron	decreased absorption of iron
	antacids	decreased absorption of the drug
Tetracycline	milk	inactivation of the drug
Thyroid hormone medications	broccoli, cauliflower, kale, kohlrabi, soybeans, Brussels sprouts, cabbage, rutabaga, turnips	decreased effectiveness of the hormone

This	can affect this	resulting in:
Alcohol	compromises magnesium	memory impairment, irritability, muscle spasm, cramps
	compromises zinc	possibly altered taste, delayed wound healing

This	can affect this	resulting in:
Alcohol (*cont'd*)	compromises vitamin B_6	poor use of iron, irritability, weakness, insomnia, rash, impaired immunity
	compromises folic acid	anemia with long-term use
	compromises thiamine	weakness, poor memory and poor attention span; pain or numbness in the legs
Aluminum-containing antacids	compromise phosphorus	confusion, muscle weakness, possible bone-thinning with long-term use
	compromise iron	lowered absorption of iron and anemia
Aspirin	compromises glucose	possible hypoglycemia with long-term use
	compromises vitamin C	poor wound healing; lowered resistance to infection
Dilantin	compromises folic acid	anemia with long-term use
Irritant laxatives	compromise potassium	low potassium condition, weakness, possible heartbeat irregularities with long-term use
	compromise calcium	muscle cramps, possible

(*continued*)

This	can affect this	resulting in:
Irritant *(cont'd)*		
		bone-thinning with long-term use
Mineral oil laxatives	compromise vitamins A, D, E, K	possible impaired immunity, bone-thinning, bleeding disorders with long-term use
Thiazide diuretics	compromise potassium	low potassium condition, weakness, possible heartbeat irregularities with long-term use
	compromise sodium	low sodium condition, weakness, coma

Bibliography

Chapter 1

Albanese, A.A. *Nutrition for the Elderly, Volume 3 of Current Topics in Nutrition & Disease.* Alan R. Liss, 1980.

Aronson, V. *A Practical Guide to Optimal Nutrition, Nutri-Plan.* John Wright PSG, 1983.

Farquhar, J.W. *The American Way of Life Need Not Be Hazardous to Your Health. The Portable Stanford.* Stanford Alumni Association, 1978.

Hamilton, E.M.N., and Whitney, E.N. *Nutrition Concepts & Controversies.* 2d ed. West Publishing Co., 1982.

Health Plus, A health promotion program of the Palm Beach County Health Department. West Palm Beach, Florida, 1984.

Chapter 2

Abraham, S. *et al.* "Relationship of Childhood Weight Status to Morbidity in Adults." *HMHA Health Reports,* March, 1971.

Albanese, A.A. *Nutrition for the Elderly, Volume 3 of Current Topics in Nutrition & Disease.* Alan R. Liss, 1980.

America in Transition: An Aging Society. Current Population Reports, Special Studies Bureau of the Census, U.S. Department of Commerce, September, 1983.

Aronson, V. *A Practical Guide to Optimal Nutrition, Nutri-Plan.* John Wright PSG, 1983.

Chanlett, E.T. *Environmental Protection,* 2nd ed. McGraw-Hill, 1979.

Developments in Aging, National Institute on Aging, National Institutes of Health, U.S. Department of Health and Human Services, 1983.

Hamilton, E.M.N., and Whitney, E.N. *Nutrition Concepts & Controversies,* 2d ed. West Publishing Co., 1982.

Hanlon, J.J., and Pickett, G.E. *Public Health Administration and Practice,* 7th ed. C.V. Mosby, 1979.

Herman, P.C., and Polivy, J. *Breaking the Diet Habit.* Basic Books, 1983.

Health Plus, A health promotion program of the Palm Beach County Health Department, West Palm Beach, Florida, 1984.

Heyden, S. *et al.* "Weight and Weight History in Relation to Cerebrovascular and Ischemic Heart Disease." *Archives of Internal Medicine,* December, 1971.

Hilts, P.J. "Life Expectancy Rises 3 Years to 74 for Men, 86 for Women." *The Washington Post,* 31 May 1983.

Kos, W.L. *et al.* "Inhibition of Host Resistance by Nutritional Hypercholesteremia." *Infection and Immunity,* November, 1979.

Last, J.M. *Maxcy-Rosenau Public Health and Preventive Medicine.* 11th ed. Appleton, Century, Croft, 1980.

Lowekopf, E.L. "Aiding the Obese to Curb Impulses to Eat." *Physician and Patient.* February, 1984.

Monro, H. "Nutritional Requirements of the Elderly." *Hospital Practice.* August, 1982.

Obesity: A Report of the Royal College of Physicians. *Journal of the Royal College of Physicians of London.* January, 1983.

Paige, D.M. *Manual of Clinical Nutrition.* Nutrition Publications, 1983.

Pizer, H. *Over Fifty-Five: Healthy & Alive.* Van Nostrand Reinhold, 1983.

Rockstein, M., and Sussman, M.L., eds. *Nutrition, Longevity and Aging.* New York: Academic Press, 1976.

Schneider, E.L., and Brody, J. Sounding Board, *The New England Journal of Medicine,* 6 October 1983.

Special Report on Aging 1982. National Institute on Aging, National Institutes of Health, U.S. Department of Health and Human Services, 1982.

Vital Statistics of the United States, 1978 Life Tables, Volume II–Section 5. National Center for Health Statistics, U.S. Department of Health and Human Services, 1980.

Yen, P.G. "A New Look at Obesity." *Geriatric Nursing.* May/June, 1983.

Chapter 3

Albanese, A.A. *Nutrition for the Elderly, Volume 3 of Current Topics in Nutrition & Disease.* Alan R. Liss, 1980.

America in Transition: An Aging Society. Current Population Reports, Special Studies Bureau of the Census, U.S. Department of Commerce, September 1983.

Biological Markers of Aging: Proceedings of the Conference on Nonlethal Biological Markers of Physiological Aging. The National Institutes of Health, U.S. Department of Health and Human Services, April, 1982.

Busse, E.W. "Eating in Late Life: Physiologic and Psychologic Factors." *New York State Journal of Medicine,* August, 1980.

Farquhar, J.W. *The American Way of Life Need Not Be Hazardous to Your Health. The Portable Stanford.* Stanford Alumni Association, 1978.

Hamilton, E.M.N., and Whitney, E.N. *Nutrition Concepts & Controversies.* 2d ed. West Publishing Co., 1982.

Morgan, B.L.G. *The Lifelong Nutrition Guide.* Prentice-Hall, 1983.

Neuhaus, R., and Neuhaus, R. *Successful Aging.* New York: John Wiley & Sons, 1982.

Paige, D.M. *Manual of Clinical Nutrition.* Nutrition Publications, 1983.

Shock, N.W. "The Role of Nutrition in Aging." *Journal of the American College of Nutrition.* December, 1981.

Special Report on Aging 1982. National Institute on Aging, National Institutes of Health, U.S. Department of Health and Human Services, 1982.

Vitale, J.J. "Impact of Nutrition on Immune Disease Function." *Advances in Human Clinical Nutrition,* John Wright PSG, 1982.

Chapter 4

Albanese, A.A. *Nutrition for the Elderly, Volume 3 of Current Topics in Nutrition & Disease.* Alan R. Liss, 1980.

Baggs, R.B., and Miller, S.A. "Defect in Resistance to Salmonella Typhimurium in Iron-Deficient Rats." *The Journal of Infectious Diseases.* October, 1974.

Bailey, L.B. *et al.* "Vitamin B_{12} Status of Elderly Persons from Low-income Households." *Journal of the American Geriatrics Society,* 28: 1980.

Bowman, B.B., and Rosenberg, I.H. "Assessment of the Nutritional Status of the Elderly." *The American Journal of Clinical Nutrition,* May, 1982.

Caggula, A.W. *et al.* "The Multiple Risk Factor Intervention Trial IV: Intervention on Blood Lipids." *Preventive Medicine,* 10: 1981.

Caloric, Nutrient and Food Intakes of Persons Ages 1–74 Years: United States, 1971–74 and 1976–80. Vital and Health Statistics, Series II, National Center for Health Statistics, U.S. Department of Health and Human Services, 1984.

Deutsch, R.M. *The New Nuts Among the Berries: How Nutrition Nonsense Captured America.* Bull Publishing, 1979.

Developments in Aging. National Institute on Aging, The National Institutes of Health, U.S. Department of Health and Human Services, 1983.

Diet, Nutrition and Cancer. Assembly of Life Sciences, National Research Council. National Academy Press, 1982.

"Excess Selenium Found Harmful CDC Reports." *American Medical News,* 20 April 1984.

Garry, P.J. *et al.* "Nutritional Status in a Healthy Elderly Population: Vitamin C." *The American Journal of Clinical Nutrition,* August, 1982.

Goodson, J.D. "Reducing the Risk of Fracture in Postmenopausal Women," presented at the course Primary Care Internal Medicine: Principles & Practice, Harvard Medical School, October 31–November 4, 1983.

Feldman, E.B., ed. *Nutrition in the Middle and Later Years.* John Wright PSG, 1983.

Hamilton, E.M.N., and Whitney, R.N. *Nutrition Concepts & Controversies.* 2d ed. West Publishing Co., 1982.

"Implications of Vitamin Use," *FDA Drug Bulletin,* November, 1983.

Kannel, W.B. *et al.* "Cholesterol in Prediction of Coronary Disease: New Perspectives Based on the Framingham Study." *Archives of Internal Medicine,* 90: 1979.

Keys, A. *Seven Counties: A Multivariate Analysis of Death and Coronary Heart Disease.* Cambridge, Mass.: Harvard University Press, 1980.

Lewis, J.S. "Vitamin C Status of Healthy Elderly Persons" (letter). *American Journal of Clinical Nutrition,* 37 (2): 1983.

Mitra, M.L. "Confusional States in Relation to Vitamin Deficiencies in the Elderly." *The Journal of the American Geriatrics Society,* 19 (6): 1971.

Morgan, B.L.G. *The Lifelong Nutrition Guide.* New York: Prentice-Hall, 1983.

Nutrition Canada. Nutrition Canada National Survey, Ottawa: Information Canada, 1983.

Nutrition and Vitamins. Medical Reference Library, Facts on File, 1983.

"Overdosing on B_6," *The Harvard Medical School of Health Letter,* December, 1983.

Paige, D.M. *Manual of Clinical Nutrition.* Nutrition Publications, 1983.

Pryor, W. "Free Radical Biology: Xenobiotics, Cancer and Aging." *Annals of the New York Academy of Sciences,* 1982.

Riggs, B.L. *et al.* "Effect of Fluoride/Calcium Regimen on Vertibral Fracture Occurrence in Post-menopausal Osteoporosis." *The New England Journal of Medicine,* 306: 1982.

Rivlin, R.S. "Nutrition and the Health of the Elderly." *Archives of Internal Medicine,* June, 1983.

Rockstein, M., and Sussman, M.L., eds. *Nutrition, Longevity and Aging.* New York: Academic Press, Inc., 1976.

Rogers, A.E. "Induction by Dimethylhydrizine of Intestinal Carcinoma in Normal Rats and Rats Fed High or Low Levels of Vitamin A." *Cancer Research,* May, 1973.

Rudman, D., and Williams, P.J. "Megadose Vitamins: Use and Misuse." *The New England Journal of Medicine,* 25 August 1983.

Schaumburg, H. *et al.* "Sensory Neuropathy from Pyridoxine Abuse." *The New England Journal of Medicine,* 25 August 1983.

Shock, N.W. "The Role of Nutrition in Aging." *Journal of the American College of Nutrition,* December, 1981.

Stare, F.J., and Aronson, V. *Dear Dr. Stare: What Should I Eat? A Guide to Sensible Nutrition.* George F. Stickley, 1982.

Stollerman, G.H., ed. *Advances in Internal Medicine,* Vols. 28 and 29. Yearbook Medical Publishers, 1984.

Tufts University Diet and Nutrition Letter, September, 1983.

Turnland, J. *et al.,* "Zinc, Copper, and Iron Balance in Elderly Men." *The American Journal of Clinical Nutrition,* December, 1981.

Vitale, J.J. "Impact of Nutrition on Immune Disease Function." *Advances in Human Clinical Nutrition.* John Wright PSG, 1982.

Weinginger, J., and Briggs, G.M., eds. *Nutrition Update,* Vol. 1. New York: John Wiley & Sons, 1983.

Willett, W.C., and MacMahon, B. "Diet and Cancer—An Overview, First of Two Parts." *The New England Journal of Medicine,* 8 March 1984.

Willett, W.C. *et al.* "Relation of Serum Vitamins A and E and Carotenoids to the Risk of Cancer." *The New England Journal of Medicine,* 16 February 1984.

Yearlick, E.S. *et al.* "Nutritional Status of the Elderly: Dietary and Biochemical Findings." *Journal of Gerontology,* 35: 1980.

Young, E. "Nutrition, Aging and the Aged." *Medical Clinics of North America,* 1983.

Chapter 5

Albanese, A.A. *et al.* "Effect of Calcium Supplementation of Serum Cholesterol, Calcium, Phosphorus and Bone Density of 'Normal, Healthy' Elderly Females." *Nutrition Reports International,* August, 1973.

"Dietary Goals for the United States," Select Committee on Nutrition and Human Needs, United States Senate, December, 1977.

Fried, E.D. "Salt, Volume, and the Prevention of Hypertension." *Circulation,* 53: 1976.

Heany, R.P. "Calcium Intake Requirement and Bone Mass in the Elderly." *Journal of Lab and Clinical Medicine,* September, 1982.

Isselbacher, K.J. *et al.,* eds. *Harrison's Principles of Internal Medicine.* 9th ed. New York: McGraw-Hill, 1980.

Lipid Research Clinics Program. "The Lipids Research Clinics Coronary Primary Prevention Trial Results: The Relationship of Reduction in Incidence of Coronary Disease to Cholesterol Lowering." *Journal of the American Medical Association,* 20 January 1984.

Podell, R.N. "Coronary Disease Prevention Proof of the Anticholesterol Pudding." *Postgraduate Medicine,* 1 May 1984.

Punsar, S. *et al.* "Coronary Heart Disease and Drinking Water." *Journal of Chronic Disease,* 28: 1975.

Resin, E. *et al.* "Effect of Weight Loss Without Salt Restriction on the Reduction of Blood Pressure." *The New England Journal of Medicine,* 298: 1978.

Science and Medicine 1983. Proceedings of a symposium by The College of Physicians and Surgeons and Columbia University, Anaheim, CA., 13 November 1983.

Sharret, Q.R., and Feinlieb, M. "Water Constituents and Trace Elements in Relation to Cardiovascular Disease." *Preventive Medicine,* 4: 1975.

Vitale, J., "Impact of Nutrition on Immune Disease Function." *Advances in Human Clinical Nutrition,* John Wright PSG, 1982.

Williams, R.R. *et al.* "Cancer Incidence by Levels of Cholesterol." *Journal of the American Medical Association,* 16 January 1981.

Chapter 6

Albanese, A.A. *Nutrition for the Elderly, Volume 3 of Current Topics in Nutrition & Disease.* Alan R. Liss, 1980.

"A Critique of Low-Carbohydrate Ketogenic Weight Reduction Regimens: A Review of Dr. Atkins' Diet Revolution." The American Medical Association Council on Foods and Nutrition, *Journal of the American Medical Association,* 4 June 1973.

Berland, T. *Rating the Diets.* Consumer Guide, 1983 ed., Signet Publications International, 1983.

Blenz, E.R., and Stein, J.S. "Obesity and Fad Diets." *Controversies in Nutrition,* Vol. 2. Churchill Livingstone, 1981.

"Block Starch or Walk Around the Block." *Harvard Medical School Health Letter,* October, 1982.

Dieting: An American Tradition. AMI Pharmacy Management Series, September, 1983.

Feldman, E.B., ed. *Nutrition in the Middle and Late Years.* John Wright PSG, 1983.

Food 2, a publication of The American Dietetics Association in cooperation with the U.S. Department of Agriculture, 1982.

Goodkind, M. "The Forgotten Ingredient." *Stanford Medicine,* Fall, 1983.

Hamilton, E.M.N., and Whitney, E.N. *Nutrition Concepts & Controversies,* 2d ed. West Publishing Co., 1982.

Mirkin, G., and Shore, R.N. "The Beverly Hills Diet: Dangers of the Newest Weight Loss Fad." *Journal of the American Medical Association,* 246: 1981.

"Mild High Blood Pressure: Getting It Down Without Drugs." *Harvard Medical School Health Letter,* August, 1983.

Mueller, S.M. "Phenylpropanolamine, A Nonprescription Drug with Potentially Fatal Side Effects" (letter). *The New England Journal of Medicine,* 17 March 1983.

Paige, D.M. *Manual of Clinical Nutrition.* Nutrition Publications, 1983.

Rivlin, R.S. "Vitamins and Minerals Related to Illness: A Cornell Postgraduate Course," Cornell University Medical College, William Douglas McAdams, Inc., 1982.

Saltzman, M.B. "Phenylpropanolamine" (letter). *The New England Journal of Medicine,* 9 February 1984.

Stare, F.J., and Aronson, V. *Dear Dr. Stare: What Should I Eat? A Guide to Sensible Nutrition.* George F. Stickley, 1982.

Stare, F.J., and McWilliams, M. *Nutrition for Good Health.* George F. Stickley, 1982.

Willis, J. "Diet Books Sell But . . ." *FDA Consumer,* March, 1982.

Chapter 10

Alcoholics Anonymous, 3d ed. AA World Services, 1976.

Farquhar, J.W. "The American Way of Life Need Not Be Hazardous to Your Health." *The Portable Stanford.* Stanford Alumni Association, 1978.

Hamilton, E.M.N., and Whitney, E.N. *Nutrition Concepts & Controversies,* 2d ed. West Publishing Co., 1982.

Health Plus, a health promotion program of the Palm Beach County Health Department, West Palm Beach, Florida, 1984.

Paige, D.M. *Manual of Clinical Nutrition.* Nutrition Publications, 1983.

Stare, F.J., and Aronson, V. *Dear Dr. Stare: What Should I Eat? A Guide to Sensible Nutrition.* George F. Stickley, 1982.

Stare, F.J., and McWilliams, M. *Nutrition for Good Health.* George F. Stickley, 1982.

Chapter 11

Aronson, V. *A Practical Guide to Optimal Nutrition, Nutri-Plan.* John Wright PSG, 1983.

"Calcium Blockers and Diet Calcium." *Harvard Medical School Health Letter,* April, 1984.

"Calcium Supplements." *Harvard Medical School Health Letter,* November, 1983.

Deutsch, R.M. *The New Nuts Among the Berries: How Nutrition Nonsense Captured America.* Bull Publishing, 1979.

"FDA Finds No Aspartame Effect." *American Medical News,* 3 February 1984.

"Hair Analysis: Another Way to Get Scalped." *Harvard Medical School Health Letter,* March, 1984.

Hamilton, E.M.N., and Whitney, E.N. *Nutrition Concepts & Controversies,* 2d ed. West Publishing Co., 1982.

"The Laxative Effect of Some Diet Foods." *Harvard Medical School Health Letter,* April, 1980.

Paige, D.M. *Manual of Clinical Nutrition.* Nutrition Publications, 1983.

Physicians Desk Reference, 4th ed. Medical Economics Company, Barnhart, 1983.

Pizer, H. *Over Fifty-Five: Healthy & Alive.* Van Nostrand Reinhold, 1983.

Stare, F.J., and Aronson, V. *Dear Dr. Stare: What Should I Eat? A Guide to Sensible Nutrition.* George F. Stickley, 1982.

Stare, F.J., and McWilliams, M. *Nutrition for Good Health.* George F. Stickley, 1982.
"Three Unproven Medical Treatments." *Harvard Medical School Health Letter,* January, 1983.
"Will It Make Angina Worse? No." *Harvard Medical School Health Letter,* January, 1984.
Zeisel, S., "The Effects of Dietary Components on Brain Function." *Advances in Human Clinical Nutrition.* John Wright PSG, 1982.

Chapter 12

Adams, C.F. The Nutritive Value of American Foods in Common Units, Agriculture Handbook #456. Washington, D.C.: Government Printing Office, 1975.
Adams, C.F., and Richardson, M. Nutritive Value of Foods, Home and Garden Bulletin #72. Washington, D.C.: Government Printing Office, 1981.
Aronson, V. *A Practical Guide to Optimal Nutrition, Nutri-Plan.* John Wright PSG, 1983.
Bordia, A. "Effect of Garlic on Blood Lipids in Patients with Coronary Heart Disease." *The American Journal of Clinical Nutrition,* October, 1981.
"Diet, Nutrition and Cancer," Assembly of the Life Sciences, National Research Council, National Academy Press, 1982.
"Consumers' Guide to Fat: Cholesterol-Controlled Food Products." Los Angeles Branch, The American Heart Association, 1978.
Farquhar, J.W. "The American Way of Life Need Not Be Hazardous to Your Health." *The Portable Stanford.* Stanford Alumni Association, 1978.
Hamilton, E.M.N., and Whitney, E.N. *Understanding Nutrition.* West Publishing Co., 1977.
Health Plus, a health promotion program of the Palm

Beach County Health Department, West Palm Beach, Florida, 1984.

Kritchevsky, D. *et al.* "Isocaloric, Isogravic Diets in Rats III. Effects of Nonnutritive Fiber (Alfalfa or Cellulose) on Cholesterol Metabolism." *Nutrition Reports International,* May, 1974.

Paige, D.M *Manual of Clinical Nutrition,* Nutrition Publications, 1983.

Paul, A.A., and Southgate, D.A.T. *McCance & Widdowson's The Composition of Foods.* 4th ed., Medical Research Council, Special Report #297, Her Majesty's Stationery Office, London, 1978.

Morgan, B.L.G. *The Lifelong Nutrition Guide.* New York: Prentice-Hall, 1983.

Stare, F.J., and Aronson, V. *Dear Dr. Stare: What Should I Eat? A Guide to Sensible Nutrition.* George F. Stickley, 1982.

Stare, F.J., and McWilliams, M. *Nutrition for Good Health.* George F. Stickley, 1982.

Chapter 13

Aronson, V. *A Practical Guide to Optimal Nutrition, Nutri-Plan.* John Wright PSG, 1983.

Columbia University Nutrition and Health Letter, Vol. 5; 3, 1983.

Deutsch, R.M. *The New Nuts Among the Berries: How Nutrition Nonsense Captured America.* Bull Publishing, 1979.

Farquhar, J.W. "The American Way of Life Need Not Be Hazardous to Your Health." *The Portable Stanford.* Stanford Alumni Association, 1978.

"Fast Food and the American Diet." A report by the American Council on Science and Health, Summit, N.J., April, 1983.

Hall, R.H. "Safe at the Plate." *Nutrition Today,* November/December, 1977.

Halpern, S.L., ed. *Quick Reference Guide to Clinical Nutrition.* J.B. Lippincott, 1979.

"Healthy People." The Surgeon General's Report on Health Promotion and Disease Prevention. U.S. Department of Health, Education and Welfare, PHS Publication 79-55071A, 1979.

Health Plus, a health promotion program of the Palm Beach County Health Department, West Palm Beach, Florida, 1984.

Information provided by the Florida Department of Health and Rehabilitative Services, in the Health Promotion Risk Reduction Program.

"The Modern American Food Supply: Is It Hazardous to Our Health?" A report by the American Council on Science and Health. *Nutrition Issues,* 18 May 1982.

Pizer, H. *Over Fifty-Five: Healthy & Alive.* Van Nostrand Reinhold, 1983.

"Of Mice & Men: The Benefits of Limitations of Animal Cancer Tests." A report by the American Council on Science and Health, May, 1984.

Rhodes, M.E. "The 'Natural' Food Myth." *The Sciences,* The New York Academy of Sciences, May/June, 1979.

Sorenson, A.W., and Ford, M.L. "Diet and Health for Senior Citizens: Workshops for the Health Team." *The Gerentologist,* 21: 1981.

Stare, F.J., and Aronson, V. *Dear Dr. Stare: What Should I Eat? A Guide to Sensible Nutrition.* George F. Stickley, 1982.

Stare, F.J., and McWilliams, M. *Nutrition for Good Health.* George F. Stickley, 1982.

Chapter 14

"After Your Heart Attack (Or Before)," *Harvard Medical School Health Letter,* April, 1982.

Blaun, R. "Exercise: The Versatile Medicine of Choice." *Medical Month,* February, 1984.

Diabetes '84. Newsletter of the American Diabetes Association, Spring, 1984.

"The Endorphins—The Body's Own Opiates," *Harvard Medical School Health Letter,* January, 1983.

"Is There Life After Jogging?" *Harvard Medical School Health Letter,* April, 1982.

Keeler, R.O. *Pep Up Your Life, A Fitness Book for Seniors,* M-10094a, The Travelers Insurance Companies, Hartford, Connecticut, 1978.

"Once Again, It's the Tortoise!" *Harvard Medical School Health Letter,* April, 1984.

Paffanberger, R.S. Jr., and Hale, W.E. "Work Activity and Coronary Heart Mortality," *The New England Journal Of Medicine,* Vol. 292, 545–550, 1975.

Sachdeo, S.K. *et al.* "Exercise in the Treatment of Diabetes Mellitus." *Practical Diabetology,* January/February, 1983.

Shephard, R.J. "Testing for Fitness in the Routine Physical." *Diagnosis,* January, 1984.

Chapter 15

"A Leisurely Look at Stress." *Harvard Medical School Health Letter,* October, 1979.

Benson, H. *et al.* "The Relaxation Response." Medical Clinics of North America, October, 1979.

Brecher, E.M. *et. al. Love, Sex and Aging, A Consumers Union Report.* Little, Brown and Company, 1984.

Comfort, A. *The Joy of Sex.* New York: Fireside, Simon & Schuster, 1972.

Comfort, A. *More Joy of Sex.* New York: Fireside, Simon & Schuster, 1974.

Renshaw, D. "Sex and the Senior Citizen." *Medical Times,* December, 1979.

"Report of the Committee on Stress, Strain and Heart Disease." The American Heart Association, *Circulation,* May, 1977.

Rosch, P.J. "Effects of Stress on the Cardiovascular System." *Physician & Patient,* November, 1983.

Chapter 16

Albanese, A.A. *Nutrition for the Elderly, Volume 3 of Current Topics in Nutrition & Disease.* Alan R. Liss, 1980.

"An Update on the Cancer-Cholesterol Connection." *Harvard Medical School Health Letter,* October, 1981.

Arbeter, A. *et al.* "Nutrition and Infection." Federation Proceedings, July/August, 1971.

Alderman, M.H. "Mild Hypertension: New Light on Old Clinical Controversy." *American Journal of Medicine,* Vol. 69, 1980.

Barice, E.J. "Considerations for Hypertension Screening and Treatment." Address before the Florida Public Health Association, 18 March 1981.

Developments in Aging. National Institute on Aging, National Institutes of Health, U.S. Department of Health and Human Services, 1983.

Diet, Nutrition and Cancer. Assembly of Life Sciences, National Research Council. National Academy Press, 1982.

"Dietary and Pharmacologic Therapy for the Lipid Risk Factors." Council Report, *Journal of the American Medical Association,* 14 October 1983.

Farquhar, J.W. "The American Way of Life Need Not Be Hazardous to Your Health." *The Portable Stanford.* Stanford Alumni Association, 1978.

Freis, E.D. "Should Mild Hypertensives Be Treated?" *New England Journal of Medicine,* 306: 1982.

Helgelend, A. "Treatment of Mild Hypertension: A Five-Year Controlled Drug Trial: The Oslo Study." *American Journal of Medicine,* Vol. 69, 1980.

"Hypertension Detection and Followup Program, Cooperative Group." *Journal of the American Medical Association,* Vol. 242, 1979.

Kannel, W.B. "Meaning of the Downward Trend in Cardiovascular Mortality." *Journal of the American Medical Association,* 12 February 1982.

Kannel, W.B. "Some Lessons in Cardiovascular Epidemiology from Framingham." *The American Journal of Cardiology,* 37: 1976.

Last, J.M. *Maxcy-Rosenau Public Health and Preventive Medicine,* 11th ed. Appleton, Century, Croft, 1980.

Monro, H. "Nutritional Requirements of the Elderly." *Hospital Practice,* August, 1982.

Morgan, B.L.G. *The Lifelong Nutrition Guide.* Prentice-Hall, 1983.

Nutrition Action, a publication of The Center for Science in the Public Interest, May, 1984.

"Nutrition and Blood Pressure Control." Annals of Internal Medicine, May, 1983.

Paige, D.M. *Manual of Clinical Nutrition.* Nutrition Publications, 1983.

Rivlin, R.S. "Nutrition and the Health of the Elderly." Archives of Internal Medicine, June, 1983.

Rowe, J.W. "Altered Blood Pressure." *Health and Disease in Old Age.* Little, Brown and Company, 1982.

Schoenberger, J.A. "The Downward Trend in Cardiovascular Mortality: Challenge and Opportunity for the Practitioner." *Journal of the American Medical Association,* 12 February 1982.

Shils, M.E. "Diet and Nutrition as Modifying Factors in Tumor Development." *Medical Clinics of North America,* September, 1979.

Special Reports on Aging 1982. National Institute on

Aging, National Institutes of Health, U.S. Department of Health and Human Services, 1982.

Toth, P.J., and Horwitz, R.I. "Conflicting Clinical Trials and the Uncertainty of Treating Mild Hypertension." *The American Journal of Medicine,* 75: 1983.

"Untreated Mild Hypertension." A report by the Management Committee of the Australian Therapeutic Trial in Mild Hypertension, *Lancet,* January, 1982.

"The War on Cancer—Where Do We Stand?" *Harvard Medical School Health Letter,* April, 1982.

Willet, W.C., and MacMahon, B. "Diet and Cancer—An Overview, First of Two Parts." *The New England Journal of Medicine,* 8 March 1984.

Willet, W.C. *et al.* "Relation of Serum Vitamins A and E and Carotenoids to the Risk of Cancer." *The New England Journal of Medicine,* 16 February 1984.

Vitale, J.J. "Impact of Nutrition on Immune Disease Function." *Advances in Human Nutrition.* John Wright PSG, 1982.

Appendix

Albanese, A.A. *Nutrition for the Elderly, Volume 3 of Current Topics in Nutrition & Disease.* Alan R. Liss, 1980.

"The Medical Letter Handbook of Drug Interactions 1983." *The Medical Letter,* 1983.

"The Medical Letter on Drugs and Therapeutics, Drug Interactions Update." *The Medical Letter,* 3 February 1984.

Morgan, B.L.G. *The Lifelong Nutrition Guide.* Prentice-Hall, 1983.

Winick, M. "Drug–Nutrient Interaction in the Elderly." An Editorial, Columbia University Health and Nutrition Newsletter, Vol. 3, 1981.

Acknowledgments

No book is an island: The Palm Beach Diet was a team effort from the start.

First we wholeheartedly thank Brian Morgan, Ph.D., assistant professor of Nutrition, Institute of Human Nutrition, College of Physicians and Surgeons, Columbia University, New York. His vast and ready knowledge of food and health contributed enormously to the authority of the Palm Beach Diet. As our technical consultant, Dr. Morgan analyzed and, in some cases, amended the nutritional profile of our original diet plans.

We thank Joseph J. Eller, M.D., of Palm Beach, author of this book's foreword, for believing in the need for an authoritative book of this nature and for his support, extensive research and valuable suggestions. Dr. Eller also enlisted the advice of several leading medical authorities on our behalf: We remain fondly grateful.

Glenn Cowley and Al Lowman were the first to see—and help shape—a book from it all. We salute their foresight.

Prominent Florida medical authorities Carl Brumback, M.D., and Jim Howell, M.D., provided confidence and inspiration. On the West Coast, John W. Farquhar, M.D., director of the Center for Research on Disease

Prevention, Stanford University, lent an ear to our ideas and volunteered helpful suggestions. His piece, "The American Way of Life Need Not Be Hazardous to Your Health" (Stanford Alumni Association), and the Health-Plus Program of the Palm Beach County Health Department, provided many excellent concepts and ideas used in this book.

A number of talented people made the production of a long and complex manuscript possible. We appreciate the long hours logged by friend and cook extraordinaire Susan Sarao, a food editor for *Cuisine* magazine; Susan brought some of our good, but basic, menus around right. We were delighted to work with Karl Ronaszeki, executive chef at The Breakers, Palm Beach, toward a collection of menus for gourmet dieters. It was a pleasure to work, too, with Frederic Hills, vice president and senior editor, Simon and Schuster; his enthusiasm and keen judgment were warmly received. And while the sun shone in the South, the typewriter clicked in the North—to the able and unflustered fingers of Debra Lennon. Thanks, Deb, for your efforts.

Moral support issued from several corners. Tom Purcell, M.D., and Dee Clauss of Palm Beach filled in and filed opinions. Fleetwood in Palm Beach and Bob in Connecticut helped keep busy coauthors from coming unglued. Thanks for soothing the way. And to Betty and Bill, and Lucille and Malcolm—our parents in their prime: This, with love and deep appreciation, is the book we wrote for you.

About the Authors

E. JOAN BARICE lives in Palm Beach, Florida, where she is in private practice in internal and preventive medicine. Formerly the Assistant Director of the Palm Beach County Health Department, she received her M.D. from Stanford University Medical School and her Master's in Public Health from the Harvard School of Public Health. Dr. Barice is Board Certified in Preventive Medicine and Internal Medicine. In 1984 she was voted the Outstanding Professional Woman of Palm Beach County by the Executive Women of the Palm Beaches.

KATHLEEN JONAH is a freelance writer who specializes in health and personal issues. She's a Contributing Editor of *Self* and former Health and Beauty Editor of British *Cosmopolitan.* Her work has appeared in *Vogue, Harper's Bazaar, The Ladies' Home Journal,* and numerous other publications. A graduate of Cordon Bleu Cookery (London), she now lives in Connecticut.